MANAGING INFLUENZA
IN PRIMARY CARE

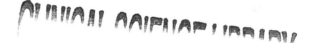

Managing Influenza in Primary Care

KARL G. NICHOLSON

MD, FRCP, FRCPath, MFPHM
Senior Lecturer in Infectious Diseases
Medical Directorate
Department of Infectious Diseases and Tropical Medicine
The Leicester Royal Infirmary
Leicester, UK

Foreword by

ARNOLD S. MONTO

**Blackwell
Science**

© 1999 by
Blackwell Science Ltd
Editorial Offices:
Osney Mead, Oxford OX2 0EL
25 John Street, London WC1N 2BL
23 Ainslie Place, Edinburgh EH3 6AJ
238 Main Street, Malden
    MA 02148 5018, USA
54 University Street, Carlton,
    Victoria 3053, Australia
10, rue Casimir Delavigne
    75006 Paris, France

Other Editorial Offices:
Blackwell Healthcare
    Communications Ltd
    Broadwalk Offices, 54 The Broadway
    Ealing, London W5 5JN

Blackwell Wissenschafts-Verlag GmbH
    Kurfürstendamm 57
    10707 Berlin, Germany

Blackwell Science KK
    MG Kodenmacho Building
    7–10 Kodenmacho Nihombashi
    Chuo-ku, Tokyo 104, Japan

DISTRIBUTORS
    Marston Book Services Ltd
    PO Box 269
    Abingdon, Oxon OX14 4YN
    (Orders: Tel: 01235 465500
                    Fax: 01235 465555)

USA
    Blackwell Science, Inc.
    Commerce Place
    350 Main Street
    Malden, MA 02148 5018
    (Orders: Tel: 800 759 6102
                          718 388 8250
                    Fax: 718 388 8255)

Canada
    Login Brothers Book Company
    324 Saulteaux Crescent
    Winnipeg, Manitoba R3J 3T2
    (Orders: Tel: 204 224 4068)

Australia
    Blackwell Science Pty Ltd
    54 University Street
    Carlton, Victoria 3053
    (Orders: Tel: 3 9347 0300
                    Fax: 3 9347 5001)

The Blackwell Science logo is a trade mark of Blackwell Science Ltd, registered at the
United Kingdom Trade Marks Registry

First published in 1999

Reprinted in 2000

ISBN 0 632 05494 8
A catalogue record for this title is available from the British Library and the Library of
Congress

Typeset by York House, London, UK
Printed by MPG Books, Bodmin, Cornwall, UK

Contents

Chapter 6: Diagnosis   48

CONTENTS

CONTENTS

Foreword

Influenza is an infectious disease full of paradoxes. It has been with us for centuries and probably millennia; the plague of Athens from the time of Hippocrates has been proposed by some to be a manifestation of influenza complicated by bacterial infection. Yet influenza is prominently listed not as an emergent (implying new), but as a re-emergent infection. This is a reflection of the capacity of the type A virus to change radically at unpredictable times and, as a consequence, to produce pandemics, spanning the world over a short period.

The world has a poor collective memory about pandemics. Interest in influenza typically wanes the longer the time since the last episode and we have not had a true pandemic for 30 years. The time appeared to have come in 1997 in a new and potentially disastrous way, with the virus of a lethal avian influenza type A/H5N1 spreading to humans in Hong Kong. No vaccine was available or could be produced. Fortunately, spread of the virus was almost exclusively from bird to human, not from human to human, and, when the poultry reservoir was eliminated, further spread ceased. This episode should be a vivid reminder of one aspect of influenza as a re-emergent problem.

On a year-to-year basis, influenza has another manifestation. It used to be thought, until modern virological techniques became commonly used, that influenza existed only when full-scale major epidemics were recognized (i.e. only episodically). This was thought to occur at a different frequency for the different types; influenza B was actually referred to as the 'quadrennial croup'. We now know that influenza occurs yearly and its annual manifestations are where it has its greatest impact on clinical practice. Thus, this problem must be faced by the practising clinician not only in years when newspaper headlines scream about the occurrence of influenza, but also in other years.

Managing Influenza in Primary Care covers this paradoxical disease in its varied manifestations. History is important because pandemics will certainly come again, so the healthcare system in general and individual physicians in particular must be prepared as best as they can. To recognize the reasons behind these events, understanding the virology is essential. In particular, without the use of some virology, perhaps, in the future, rapid diagnostic techniques, the full clinical impact of the infection cannot be understood.

Typical influenza probably represents fewer than 20% of cases. The other less typical cases may still produce the complications well recognized to occur in predictable segments of the population. This epidemiological characteristic, that individuals with various chronic conditions are likely to develop complications leading to hospitalization and sometimes death, has been the reason that current vaccination policies have been adopted. These policies have been developed to reduce the likelihood that these complications will occur, even though we know that most of the disease is seen in younger people and in families.

Why is it so appropriate that we examine influenza management at the present time? As this volume points out, after many years with no new interventions for the control of influenza, we are now at a point when new preventive and treatment approaches are on the horizon. The inactivated vaccine has been used with good effect for more than 50 years but a live attenuated influenza vaccine is now in development, which may be particularly useful in controlling morbidity in children.

Perhaps even more exciting is the impending availability of antiviral agents specific for treatment and prophylaxis of influenza. Amantadine and, in some countries, rimantadine have been available for these purposes for many years but have been underused. They also have certain limitations: they are active only against type A viruses, have side effects that can be a problem and produce resistant variants predictably.

The new class of antivirals, the neuraminidase inhibitors, are a major advance because they are equally useful against influenza A and B infection. Not only can they be used in treatment but data suggest that they are also suitable for prophylaxis. They have already been successfully shown to prevent illness over a period of weeks. In practice, they may be used more frequently in preventing spread, usually in a family, to exposed individuals from primary recognized cases of influenza. Perhaps they will also be useful in institutions such as nursing homes, which continue to be sites where influenza frequently causes outbreaks. They are likely to revolutionize the treatment of influenza because they shorten the duration of illness, allow patients to return to normal activity more quickly and appear even to prevent complications. To optimize their use, improved understanding and recognition of influenza is critical. This volume will be a great advance in achieving these ends.

Arnold S. Monto
University of Michigan
Ann Arbor, Mich., USA

Preface

Few conditions exert such an enormous toll of absenteeism, suffering, medical consultations, hospitalization, death and economic loss as influenza. Despite its widespread annual occurrence, there was, until recently, little advance in the control of influenza since the licensing of amantadine more than 30 years ago. The 1990s, however, have seen accruing evidence on the effectiveness of inactivated influenza vaccines and also the efficacy and safety of live influenza virus vaccines. Furthermore, work on the viral neuraminidase has led to potent and selective inhibitors and opened up exciting therapeutic options for the treatment and prevention of influenza. Add to this the issue of making a correct clinical diagnosis of influenza, the role of rapid sensitive laboratory diagnostic techniques, the development of near-patient testing and the possibility of a pandemic of influenza in the foreseeable future, the justification for preparing this book is evident. *Managing Influenza in Primary Care* is not intended to be a definitive textbook covering a full range of topics but rather is a succinct overview of selected material that provides quick access to relevant background and practical information for busy medical and nurse practitioners. Size limitations have not permitted the citation of the many key articles that were reviewed in preparing this book. Instead, the more investigative reader is directed – as I was – to the *Textbook of Influenza* (eds Karl G. Nicholson, Robert G. Webster and Alan J. Hay, Blackwell Science, Oxford, 1998) for more scholarly accounts by experts in each field and to Web sites (see overleaf) that can be used to keep fully up to date.

Karl G. Nicholson
Leicester Royal Infirmary
Leicester, UK

Acknowledgements

This book would not have existed without the enthusiasm, support and direction of Ellen Sarewitz and her editorial team at Blackwell Healthcare Communications. I am particularly indebted to Sarah Harrison at Blackwell Healthcare, Dr Nigel Higson and especially Dr Arnold Monto for their many helpful suggestions and encouragement. Last but not least, I acknowledge the support, understanding and tolerance provided by my wife and children.

Some useful Web sites

NIMR Influenza Bibliography:
http://www.nimr.mrc.ac.uk/Library/flu

Centers for Disease Control and Prevention – Influenza Prevention and Control: http://www.cdc.gov/ncidod/diseases/flu/fluvirus.htm

FluNet (WHO's geographical information system to monitor influenza): http://oms.b3e.jussieu.fr/flunet/

National Library of Medicine Influenza Page:
http://medlineplus.nlm.nih.gov/medlineplus/influenza.html

European Influenza Surveillance Scheme:
http://www.eiss.org/public/present.htm

European Scientific Working Group on Influenza:
http://www.eswi.org

CHAPTER 1

Pandemics in history

- Influenza causes periodic seasonal epidemics and, very occasionally, global pandemics involving many millions of people
- Sero-archaeology indicates the subtypes of influenza that have circulated in recent history and gives insight into the nature of pandemic influenza
- Clinical characteristics of pandemics are difficult to predict in advance and vary greatly
- At least four influenza pandemics have occurred this century, most recently in 1977–1978

Introduction

The existence of the highly infectious acute respiratory illness known as influenza has been recognized for over 2000 years. In classical Greece, clinical descriptions during the Great Plague of Athens (430–427 BC) indicate that staphylococcal toxic shock syndrome may have occurred as a complication. The pandemic of Spanish influenza in 1918–1920, which caused more than 20 million deaths, was referred to as the last great plague. More recently, the small but highly lethal 1997 outbreak in Hong Kong reminded us that influenza has lost none of its deadly potential.

Unlike many infectious diseases, influenza has no pathognomonic features, so a precise picture of its impact was not possible until after isolation of the viral types A (1933), B (1940) and C (1947). The discovery of the haemagglutinating properties of the virus in 1941 led to a diagnostic test, providing the means to monitor the spread and impact of influenza. However, knowledge of its characteristics – tendency for seasonality, short incubation period, rapid dissemination, respiratory and systemic features – enables us to construct a picture of influenza since ancient times.

1

Figure 1.1. History of pandemics since 1580				
Year	Affected countries	First recognized	Origin	Comments
1580	Europe, Africa, N America	Summer	Asia	
1729–1733	Europe, Russia, N & S America	Spring	Russia	Two distinct waves or two distinct epidemics; second more severe
1781–1782	Europe, China, India, N America, Russia	Autumn	Russia/ China	Two waves; second more severe
1830–1833	Europe, Russia, N America, India, China	Winter	China	Two waves; second more severe
1847–1848	Europe, Russia, N America (?)	Spring	Asia/ Russia	Some disagreement by historians: possibly not genuine pandemic
1889–1891	Global	Spring	Russia	Extensive seeding in spring and summer; winter pandemic. Later waves more severe
1900	Europe, Australia, N & S America	Not known	Not known	Little clinical illness; new virus subtype indicated by serology
1918–1920	Global	Spring	USA/ China	Two distinct phases; second more severe
1957–1958	Global	Winter/ spring	China	Two waves; second of equal or greater severity
1968–1970	Global	Summer	China	In Europe, peak 1 year after USA
1977–1978	Global	Summer	China/ Russia	
Adapted with permission from Potter CW. Chronicle of influenza pandemics. In: Nicholson KG, Webster RG, Hay AJ, eds. *Textbook of Influenza*. Oxford: Blackwell Science, 1998: 3–18.				

At least 10 pandemics of influenza-like illness have occurred since the end of the 16th century. Although perhaps not all were due to influenza, at least four pandemics have emerged during this century alone and the events in Hong Kong in 1997, when six deaths occurred among 18 people hospitalized with influenza A/H5N1 ('bird flu'), should alert us to the possibility that the next pandemic could cause as many deaths in young adults as the pandemic of 1918–1920.

Pandemic definition

The word pandemic (from the Greek *pan* meaning all and *demos* meaning people) is used to describe an epidemic that affects the whole population. Typically, several waves of infection, occurring over a few years, are needed before most of the population is infected by a new virus subtype. A pandemic is considered imminent or said to exist when the following apply.

- 'Antigenic shift' occurs, i.e. the emergence in humans of a new subtype of influenza A, which is serologically distinct from earlier viruses and could not have arisen from these viruses by mutation
- A high proportion of the population lacks immunity to the new virus
- The new virus spreads from person to person, causing disease
- The new virus spreads rapidly beyond the community in which it was first identified

That pandemic strains originate from reassortment of human and animal subtypes of influenza A is well accepted. Evidence indicates that the virus responsible for the 1918–1920 pandemic crossed the species barrier into humans probably from pigs, although it originated from birds. Occasionally, however, the genetic mutations associated with antigenic drift of influenza A can be so profound that an established subtype can behave like a novel 'pandemic' virus.

Lessons from the past

Almost all pandemics since the middle of the 19th century have been accompanied by marked increases in mortality. The pandemic of 1847–1848, which began in Russia, was no exception. During the worst 2 months, weekly deaths exceeded the average by about 60%

and deaths attributed to lung diseases showed an excess of 90%. Influenza was responsible for many hidden deaths, a phenomenon still evident today.

Sero-archaeology

By examining blood samples from people of varying ages for the presence of antibodies, we can identify whether a particular subtype of influenza circulated previously and, if so, approximately when it ceased to circulate. This type of study is known as sero-archaeology.

In 1957, specimens collected from elderly people before that year's H2 influenza pandemic were found to contain antibodies to the new pandemic virus. Elevated levels of antibody were present only in people born before 1886, suggesting that an H2 subtype of the virus may have circulated in 1847–1888.

Similarly, blood collected 10 years before the 1968 H3 pandemic from people aged at least 70 years was found to contain antibody reacting with H3 strains of horse influenza. Subsequently, in 1968, workers in Atlanta found H3 antibody in pre-pandemic sera from people born before 1896 but not later. In Holland, a steep age-related increase in the prevalence of antibodies to the Hong Kong pandemic virus was also found in people born before 1896.

Together these findings suggest that an H3 subtype of the influenza virus circulated during the 1890s and that it was almost certainly responsible for the pandemic in 1889. Lower mortality during the 1968–1970 pandemic in people over 75 years old, compared with those aged 65–74 years, supports this theory.

Sero-archaeology has been described as attempting to 'reconstruct the skeleton of a dinosaur from a few teeth and some fragments of bone'. Nonetheless, such studies have established beyond reasonable doubt that H2 and H3 subtypes circulated in human populations during both the 19th and the 20th centuries.

The pandemic of 1918–1920

The hallmarks of the 1918–1920 pandemic were its three increasingly severe waves, exceedingly high case-fatality rate, extraordinary toll on healthy young adults and obscure origin.

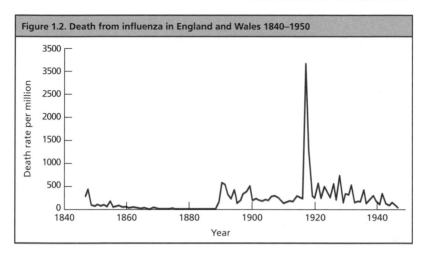

Figure 1.2. Death from influenza in England and Wales 1840–1950

The appearance of an influenza-like illness among pigs in the American Midwest in 1918 led to the discovery of the porcine influenza virus in 1931. The serological studies that followed provided clues that the 1918 pandemic had been caused by a porcine influenza virus. Subsequent sero-archaeological studies showed that antibodies to the porcine strain were present in the serum of people born before the early 1920s. In 1997, the partial sequencing of viral gene segments from lung tissue of a soldier who died from influenza in 1918 revealed a genetic similarity to porcine influenza viruses.

Perhaps because most pandemics in history originated in the Far East, historians have postulated a possible origin in China. Many labourers were migrating from China, where influenza was recorded, to North America in 1918.

During the spring outbreak, a distinctly unusual pattern of mortality from influenza and pneumonia first appeared, namely an excessive and disproportionate increase in deaths among young adults.

The pandemic virus spread rapidly, causing deaths among soldiers during the voyage to Europe in March 1918. Within 3 months, the virus had crossed the Pacific and Atlantic oceans and the first wave attacked all of the armies in Europe throughout May and June 1918. A second, killing wave, which brought a far greater incidence of serious

1

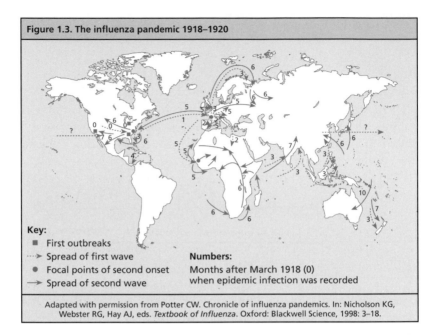

Figure 1.3. The influenza pandemic 1918–1920

Key:
- ■ First outbreaks
- ⋯▶ Spread of first wave
- ● Focal points of second onset
- ⟶ Spread of second wave

Numbers:
Months after March 1918 (0)
when epidemic infection was recorded

Adapted with permission from Potter CW. Chronicle of influenza pandemics. In: Nicholson KG, Webster RG, Hay AJ, eds. *Textbook of Influenza*. Oxford: Blackwell Science, 1998: 3–18.

complications, peaked almost simultaneously around the world that autumn. The third wave occurred in the spring of 1919.

Deaths during the pandemic were age-related and followed the W-shaped pattern noted in retrospect during the first wave. The mortality is puzzling. Although 5–14-year-olds had the highest incidence of influenza during the pandemic, they had the lowest mortality. Inexplicably, 25–40-year-olds had an intermediate incidence of influenza but the highest incidence of pneumonia and a case-fatality rate that was exceeded only by that of the very elderly (in whom the incidence of influenza-like illness was lowest). In 10 months, this 'Spanish flu' killed an estimated 20–40 million people worldwide.

The pandemic of 1957–1958

The H2N2 influenza pandemic of 1957–1958 originated in China's Kweichow province. The virus, referred to as A/Asian/57 or 'Asian flu', caused extensive infection in China during March 1957 and spread rapidly in Southeast Asia and to Japan and Australia. World Health Organization (WHO) laboratories on three continents identified the isolates as being distinct from those circulating during the previous decade. Human serological studies led to the conclusion that most of the world's population lacked antibodies to this specific subtype.

Attack rates ranged from about 20% to almost 100% in different communities worldwide, with higher rates (>50%) among schoolchildren, the institutionalized and those living in crowded conditions. During the autumn epidemic, clinical cases in England and Wales occurred in 31% of all age groups but the peak attack rate (49%) was seen in schoolchildren aged 5–14 years.

During the first wave, claimants for sickness benefit in England and Wales increased from an average of 2.5 million to 4.5 million. Nursing levels in hospitals were significantly reduced. Nearly half of the school population was absent at some time during the epidemic. Primary care practices with up to 14 000 registered patients reported seeing 50–150 cases each day. In London, the Emergency Bed Service placed nearly three times as many patients with acute respiratory disease as normal during the autumn wave.

The 1957–1958 pandemic was generally regarded, on the basis of deaths, as rather mild. An excess of 33 000 deaths occurred during the autumn wave in England and Wales, of which only 6716 were attributed to influenza. In the USA, 39 000 deaths occurred during the first wave and a further 20 000 during the second wave. Overall mortality was about 10% of that seen during the pandemic of 1918–1920.

The pandemic of 1968–1970

An outbreak of H3N2 influenza that began in China in July 1968 spread to Hong Kong, where it affected some 500 000 people. The peak incidence in Hong Kong occurred in late July, only 2 weeks after the first isolation of the A/Hong Kong virus, and the whole outbreak was over in 6 weeks. In August, the virus entered Taiwan, Singapore, Malaysia, Vietnam and the Philippines; it reached India, Australia and Japan in September. In the USA, a nationwide epidemic peaked in December 1968. Some 30–40% of the population was affected, schools had 50% absenteeism and more than 56 000 deaths were attributed to the outbreak. In Europe, the disease was considered mild, although Poland had an estimated four million cases.

The pandemic of 1977–1978

The H1N1 influenza virus that caused the 1977–1978 pandemic appeared in Anshan, northern China, in May 1977. By mid-December, all large cities in Siberia and European Russia were affected. Subsequent analysis revealed that it was identical to a virus that had caused a human epidemic in 1950. In 1978, outbreaks of infection with the prototype virus A/USSR/77 occurred throughout the New World, Europe, the Middle East and Australasia.

Because H1N1 viruses circulated before the 'Asian flu' pandemic in 1957–1958, most people over 23 years old possessed antibodies to the new virus and outbreaks of infection were confined almost entirely to children and teenagers. The highest weekly attack rates at the peak of the epidemic reached 13% in children aged 7–14 years and the illness was generally mild. Unlike the former two pandemic viruses, that of 1977–1978 failed to replace the previously circulating influenza A virus and, to this day, both H1N1 and H3N2 subtypes of influenza A and influenza B virus co-circulate in humans.

False alarms?

The A/New Jersey/76 H1N1 outbreak in 1976

A localized outbreak of porcine influenza at Fort Dix, USA, with a fatal index case, lasted from 19 January to 9 February 1976. It infected at least 230 military personnel but did not spread to the civilian population. The response in the USA included partial implementation of a programme of mass immunization.

The A/Hong Kong/97 H5N1 outbreak in 1997

In mid-May 1997, a 3-year-old boy died in the Queen Elizabeth Hospital, Hong Kong, from acute respiratory distress syndrome and Reye's syndrome. A tracheal aspirate revealed an influenza A virus that differed only slightly from that responsible for an earlier outbreak of avian influenza on three chicken farms. Six months later, 17 further cases occurred. Surveillance of markets revealed the presence of the virus in poultry. After the 18th (and final) virologically confirmed case in a human, in December 1997, slaughter of poultry was instituted. The outbreak caused six deaths among 18 cases.

Because avian viruses replicate poorly in humans and vice versa, pigs were proposed as the intermediate 'mixing vessel' for the generation of reassortants. The farming practices, bird markets and dense populations of people, pigs and ducks in southern China would facilitate interspecies transmission of virus into a porcine 'mixing vessel' and might explain why China has been the epicentre of recent pandemics. However, the finding of human–avian reassortment viruses in pigs in Italy and in humans in Holland indicates that a pandemic could also emerge as a result of genetic reassortment in Europe or North America. Direct transmission of avian strains to humans also occurs, as in the case of the 1997 H5N1 outbreak in Hong Kong.

CHAPTER 2

The influenza virus

- Influenza virus occurs in three types (A, B and C) and numerous subtypes and strains; A and B have the greatest impact on human health
- Influenza A and B have two surface glycoproteins: the haemagglutinin (HA) and the neuraminidase (NA)
- Influenza A and B constantly change their antigenic form by antigenic 'drift' and, less frequently, by antigenic 'shift' (influenza A only), when the genomes of two existing subtypes are mixed by genetic reassortment
- Reassortment allows specific vaccines to be produced, by combining the antigens from virulent isolates with attenuated virus
- Zoonotic transmission of avian and mammalian influenza occurs, thereby maintaining a global reservoir of influenza

Introduction

Influenza viruses belong to the family Orthomyxoviridae, from the Greek *myxa* meaning mucus, a reference to the special association of the viruses with mucosal surfaces. The origin of the word 'influenza' is uncertain. It is said to occur in the chronicles of a Florentine family in the 14th and 15th centuries in connection with the possible influence of the planets at times of respiratory epidemics. 'Influenza' was first used in England in 1743 to describe an illness rife throughout Europe. The French term for the illness, 'la grippe' (probably from *agripper* meaning to seize), came into use the same year.

Antigenic types and subtypes

Influenza viruses are unique among respiratory viruses in their segmented genome and great antigenic diversity. They were originally

Figure 2.1. Influenza virus

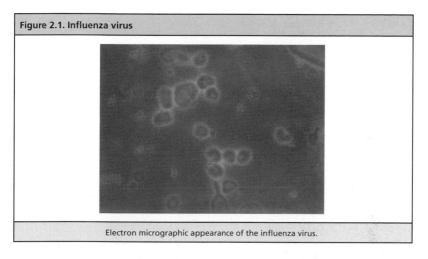

Electron micrographic appearance of the influenza virus.

classified serologically into three distinct types, A, B and C, on the basis of differences in their core proteins. Sequencing studies have confirmed this classification scheme but have shown that all influenza viruses evolved from a common ancestor.

The structures of influenza A, B and C are generally similar when visualized by electron microscopy. Most influenza viruses are spherical particles but filamentous forms can also be seen. Influenza B preparations reveal less variation in size and shape and most particles appear round. With negative staining, spikes representing the surface glycoproteins haemagglutinin (HA) and neuraminidase (NA) can be seen on the viral surface. Influenza C particles are of similar shape and size but differ in that they have a single surface glycoprotein

Influenza A viruses are further divided into subtypes depending on antigenic differences between their coating of surface glycoproteins. Fifteen subtypes of HA (H1–H15) and nine subtypes of NA (N1–N9) are now recognized for influenza A. Only one novel HA has been discovered in the past 10 years, despite extensive surveillance of influenza in humans and animals, implying that the number of HAs and NAs in nature is finite.

Influenza type A viruses of all HA and NA antigenic subtypes have been recovered from birds but only a few infect other animal species; this indicates that birds are the natural reservoirs of influenza A.

11

Influenza B is restricted to humans. The natural hosts of influenza C include humans, pigs and possibly dogs.

Epidemiological studies indicate that influenza A is responsible for periodic worldwide pandemics and frequent epidemics that are often associated with considerable morbidity and mortality. Influenza B is less frequent and is associated with a lower burden of illness overall. Influenza C is associated with sporadic, often asymptomatic infection with little or no mortality and therefore is not a public health concern.

Antigenic 'shift' and 'drift'

- **Antigenic drift:** gene mutations, especially within genes encoding the surface glycoproteins, resulting in changes in the antigenic nature of the virus
- **Antigenic shift:** reassortment of gene segments during dual infection with influenza A viruses of differing subtypes

Pandemics and epidemics arise as a result of changes in the HA that coats the influenza virus. Pandemic influenza is the outcome of antigenic 'shift', which reflects a major change in the HA and possibly NA antigens and occurs only with influenza A virus. A reassortment of gene segments during dual infection with human and avian influenza A viruses of differing subtypes has led to periodic antigenic shifts and brought into being new pandemic strains. The 1957–1958 and 1968–1970 pandemic strains of influenza were reassortants with genes from both human and avian viruses. Pig trachea contains receptors for both avian and human influenza viruses and, acting as an intermediate 'mixing vessel', can support the replication and reassortment of human and avian viruses.

Pandemics may also evolve by transmission of non-human viruses to humans without prior reassortment, as happened during the highly lethal outbreak of A/H5N1 infection in Hong Kong in 1997. Fortunately, this subtype failed to reassort in humans with a human virus and evidently did not acquire the ability to pass from human to human. Only 18 cases were reported, all of which were assumed to have passed from birds.

The occurrence of repeated outbreaks of influenza A during inter-pandemic periods is related to gene mutations, especially within genes encoding the surface glycoproteins. These result in changes in the anti-genic nature of the virus, known as antigenic 'drift', which allow the virus subtype to escape immune recognition. New strains of influenza evolve within each type and subtype of influenza at rates depending on the genetic stability of the virus and the immune pressure.

2

The surface glycoproteins

During the early 1940s, investigators noted that a suspension of influenza virus would agglutinate erythrocytes. These observations showed that the influenza virus possessed an HA and that the specific receptor for the virus was present on the surface of erythrocytes. It pro-vided a method of detecting and titrating the virus and its antibodies.

When the influenza virus and erythrocytes were warmed to 37°C, the erythrocytes dispersed but did not reagglutinate on subsequent exposure to fresh virus. However, fluid from the original mixture of virus and cells would still agglutinate fresh cells. This phenomenon suggested that the virion possesses an enzyme that destroys its own receptor. The substance cleaved from erythrocytes was subsequently identified as sialic acid (N-acetylneuraminic acid) and the receptor-destroying enzyme was called NA or sialidase.

The HA is now the primary constituent of influenza vaccine and the NA has become a major target for antiviral treatment.

Haemagglutinin

The first important function of the HA is to attach the virus to sialic acid-containing receptors on the cell surface; the virus then undergoes endocytosis, exposing the HA to a relatively low pH. The decrease in pH results in an irreversible conformational change in the HA, which is essential for fusion of the virus envelope with the cell membrane.

Cleavage of the HA precursor, HA_0, by an intracellular enzyme (endoprotease), secretory proteases and, possibly, proteases produced by certain bacteria and house-dust mites is essential for infectivity and is a major determinant of virulence. The HAs of some pathogenic avian viruses contain a series of basic amino acids at the cleavage site and are cleaved by ubiquitous endoproteases; these can give rise to high titres of infectious virus in all organs and can cause a systemic fatal disease in the bird. Although the human and avian isolates of the A/H5N1 virus in Hong Kong in 1997 possess high pathogenicity, no available evidence indicates that that virus causes systemic infection in humans. The deaths in Hong Kong appeared to be due to typical influenza complications, such as pneumonia.

The HA represents the major antigenic determinant of influenza types A and B and induces neutralizing antibodies. For survival, influenza viruses must evade immune recognition by a process of continual evolution. Human influenza viruses respond readily to immune pressure, with new variant viruses emerging with each round of replication. The ability to form variants that escape immune recognition (i.e. antigenic drift) is regarded as a further important function of the HA.

The location of glycosylation sites on the HA, and hence oligosaccharides, are of importance by masking or uncovering antigenic sites and the cleavage site. Mutations that add glycosylation sites near an antigenic site can produce virus populations that are masked immunologically (i.e. protected from immune recognition). Conversely, the removal of glycosylation sites near the HA cleavage site can enhance both cleavage and virulence of certain viruses.

Neuraminidase

The NA is the second major antigenic determinant of influenza types A and B. The viral NA is anchored in the viral envelope and projects outward from the virus. The following functions have been proposed for the enzyme activity of the NA.

- Assisting in the release of progeny virus particles from the surface of infected cells
- Preventing virus clumping so that each virion can function as an independent infectious unit
- Facilitating cleavage of HA (may thus be implicated in virulence), by modifying HA carbohydrate side chains
- Facilitating movement of virus though inhibitory mucopolysaccharides coating the respiratory tract epithelium

Evidence also suggests that viral NA is involved in virus assembly and that antigenic drift of the NA helps the virus to survive. Single amino acid sequence changes on the top of the NA head result in antigenic variants that escape immune recognition.

Virus ion channels

The M2 protein is an integral part of the envelope of influenza A. The function of M2, common to all subtypes of influenza A, is to facilitate the uncoating of the virus during its entry into cells so that its ribonucleoprotein can enter nuclei and initiate replication. This activity can be blocked in influenza A viruses by the antiviral agents amantadine and rimantadine.

Genetic reassortment

Both the A/Asian/57 H2N2 and the A/Hong Kong/68 H3N2 pandemics originated by reassortment of gene segments during co-infection of cells by a human and an avian virus. A total of 256 combinations of gene segments is possible when two different influenza viruses, each containing eight gene segments, infect the same cell simultaneously.

The phenomenon of genetic reassortment has been put to practical use, providing vaccine manufacturers with a method of producing candidate live-attenuated virus vaccines by transfer of genes from an attenuated donor virus to a virulent wild-type virus by co-infection of tissue culture cells. By this means, an attenuated cold-adapted live virus vaccine can contain the genes that encode the HA and NA from the virulent wild-type virus and genes that confer attenuation from the attenuated donor virus.

Moreover, genetic reassortment between a vaccine strain and a high-yield donor virus is used each year to produce a fast-growing virus, a high-growth reassortant, with which to manufacture inactivated vaccine.

Replication

The parasitic association of viruses with the host cell originally led to the belief that drugs that interfere with the viral life cycle would inevitably be toxic to the host. An improved understanding of viral

2

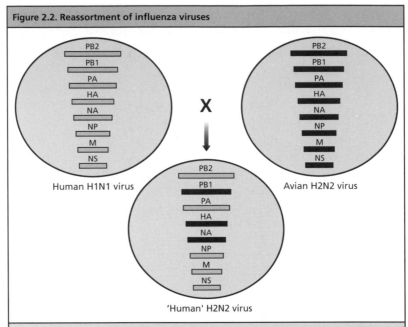

Figure 2.2. Reassortment of influenza viruses

Human H1N1 virus

X

Avian H2N2 virus

'Human' H2N2 virus

In 1957, the Asian pandemic virus acquired three gene segments (PB1, HA and NA) from the avian influenza gene pool in wild ducks and retained five other genes from the previously circulating H1N1 human strain. In 1968, the Hong Kong pandemic virus acquired two genes (PB1 and an HA coding for H3) from the avian pool and retained six genes from the H2N2 virus circulating in humans.

replication has led to the recognition that key events are unique to the virus and drugs can be targeted to the virus, inhibiting viral replication without undue toxicity to the host.

The cycle of replication in susceptible cells in the respiratory tract takes about 4–6 hours. Thereafter, virus is released for several hours before cell death and progeny virions initiate infection in adjacent cells, so that, within a short period, many cells in the respiratory tract are either infected, releasing virus or dying.

Avian influenza

Influenza viruses have been isolated from a wide range of wild and domestic bird species. The following orders all contain families from

Figure 2.3. Replication of the influenza virus

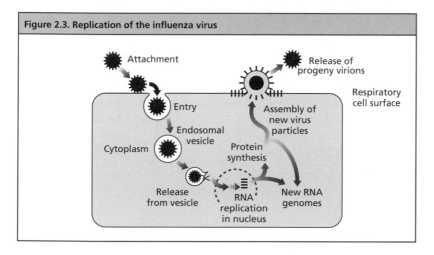

which virus has been isolated (the greatest number have been isolated from aquatic birds).

- Procellariiformes (shearwaters)
- Pelecaninformes (cormorants)
- Anseriformes (swans, geese, ducks)
- Galliformes (turkeys, quail)
- Ciconiiformes (herons, ibis)
- Gruiformes (rails, coots)
- Charadriiformes (gulls, turnstones)

Virus has also been isolated from Passeriformes (starlings, mynas) but has not been recovered from Psittacines (parrots and budgerigars).

Signs of disease

In ducks, influenza virus replicates in the gastrointestinal epithelium and is excreted at a high concentration in the faeces without causing any sign of disease. However, the disease signs associated with different avian viruses vary among species and birds are affected with varying levels of severity. Infection with most strains is completely asymptomatic, whereas a few strains can cause a rapidly fatal disease (fowl plague). Features of infection may include cyanosis of the combs (fleshy crest) and wattles (fleshy throat), respiratory signs, ruffled feathers, diarrhoea and central nervous system (CNS) involvement.

Transmission and persistence of virus in nature

Influenza viruses are found in wild ducks in the northern hemisphere mostly during August and September. Birds hatched in the spring provide a large susceptible population. Infection spreads rapidly, with up to 30% of juvenile birds shedding virus as they congregate in marshalling areas before migration.

Harsh winter conditions provide optimal conditions for virus survival. Laboratory studies indicate that virus can survive in faecal material for 7 days at 20°C, for as long as 30 days at 4°C and for even longer when frozen. However, viable virus has not been detected in lake water tested during the winter months. Moreover, because the predominant subtype of influenza varies from flyway to flyway and from year to year, influenza must be perpetuated in wild ducks by other means.

One possibility is that the virus circulates at a low level throughout the winter. Alternatively, infection could be perpetuated by other avian species living along the migratory pathways and wild ducks could become infected during their migration. Influenza viruses have been recovered from various shore birds and the influenza gene pool in shore birds is common with that in ducks, suggesting the possibility of transmission between the different avian species. Evidence suggests transmission of influenza virus from migrating ducks to domestic poultry.

Transmission to other animals

Evidence shows that birds can transmit influenza virus to humans and other animals.

- **Humans:** avian influenza viruses belonging to the H7 and H10 subtypes have been recovered from eye swabs from two people with conjunctivitis. The first had contact with ducks and the second with an infected seal that sneezed into the person's face and right eye. H5N1 virus was recovered from 18 people hospitalized with influenza in Hong Kong in 1997. Serological surveys indicate that several hundred additional cases of human H5 influenza may have occurred. Sero-surveys in southern China reveal that rural dwellers in the 'influenza epicentre' contain antibody to avian subtypes H4 to H13

- **Horses:** an outbreak of H3N8 influenza among horses in northeastern China in 1989, which caused up to 20% mortality among some herds, was due to a virus not previously found in China. Antigenic and molecular studies suggest an avian origin
- **Pigs:** porcine influenza viruses possessing avian genes were first detected in Europe in 1979. Molecular studies of the internal genes of 10 H1N1 and 11 H3N2 porcine influenza viruses isolated in Italy between 1992 and 1995 showed them to be of avian origin
- **Mink:** during 1994, an epizootic of H10N7 influenza occurred on coastal mink farms in southern Sweden. One hundred thousand mink were affected, with 3000 deaths. Seabirds are believed to have transmitted the virus when trying to eat the food in the mink cages
- **Whales:** influenza A viruses belonging to the H1 and H13 subtypes have been recovered from the lungs and other organs of whales. Genetic analysis showed that the isolates were related to recent gull and tern isolates. The available evidence suggests independent transmission from birds rather than continual circulation in whales
- **Seals:** infections with H3, H4 and H7 subtypes have been identified

Porcine influenza

In 1918, during the pandemic of human influenza in the Midwest of the USA, an American vet, J. S. Koen, first noted an epizootic of respiratory illness in which many thousands of pigs died. There were reports at the time of farmers getting the disease from pigs and vice versa. Koen called it 'influenza' and thereafter outbreaks were noted each autumn. In 1931, Richard Shope showed that bacteria-free filtrates of infective material produced a mild illness when inoculated intranasally into pigs and that full-blown disease occurred when pigs were infected with both the filtrate and the bacterium *Haemophilus influenzae suis*.

Sero-archaeological studies carried out in the 1950s and 1970s revealed high levels of antibody to porcine influenza in the sera of people born before 1921. In 1997, the partial sequencing of the viral gene segments from the lung tissue of a soldier who died from influenza in 1918 revealed close genetic similarity to early porcine influenza strains, corroborating the sero-archaeological findings. There have been occasional reports of the introduction of porcine H1N1 influenza into the human population and at least 11 deaths have been reported since 1974, when a porcine virus was first isolated from a human.

The domestic pig is the only species known to support the growth of viruses of both human and avian origin and, for this reason, is considered to be a 'mixing vessel' for the reassortment of viruses from both species. H1N1 and H3N2 are the only subtypes of influenza A that are consistently recovered from pigs.

Human-like influenza H3N2 viruses were first isolated from pigs during a human epidemic in Taiwan. Since then, they have been recovered from pigs in several parts of the world, including Europe. Two aberrant H3N2 viruses were detected from two young children in separate geographical regions in Holland during the 1992–1993 influenza season. The serological and genetic studies that followed confirmed that they were human–avian reassortants that were circulating in European pigs.

The frequency of transmission of porcine H1N1 and H3N2 viruses to humans was tested by examination of 123 human sera in Italy. The findings suggest that approximately 20% of people less than 20 years old who had contact with pigs may have been infected with porcine H3N2 influenza viruses containing avian-derived genes. These observations alert us to the possibility of a European epicentre for the next pandemic and indicate that pigs should be surveyed continuously for evidence of novel virus reassortants.

Equine influenza

Two subtypes of influenza, H7N7 and H3N8, have formed stable lineages in horses. H7N7 virus has not been isolated since the early 1980s but H3N8 virus causes equine influenza in many parts of the world. Sero-archaeological studies suggest that an H3N8 virus may have circulated in humans towards the end of the last century. However, genetic analyses indicate that equine and human H3 HAs emerged independently from avian ancestors.

2

Strains of influenza are identified on the basis of type (i.e. A, B or C), host of origin (e.g. avian, porcine), geographical site of virus isolation (e.g. Asian, Hong Kong), serial number, year of isolation and, for influenza A viruses, subtypes of HA and NA antigens.

CHAPTER 3

Epidemiology

3

- Transmission of influenza occurs by inhalation of microdroplets, followed by a 4–6-hour replication cycle and profuse viral shedding
- Shedding may precede symptoms by 1–2 days, leading to potentially high attack rates
- Seasonal epidemics are common in many countries, with the influenza season typically occurring during the winter
- Since 1977, influenza A/H3N2, A/H1N1 and B strains have been co-circulating, with one strain usually predominating

Transmission

Influenza is spread by virus-laden respiratory secretions. Most infections appear to be transmitted by droplets several micrometres in diameter that are expelled during coughing and sneezing, rather than by fine droplet nuclei. The human infectious dose is estimated to be 0.6 to 3 tissue culture infectious doses after small-particle aerosol exposure and about 100 times greater for virus administered by nosedrops. Pathological evidence suggests initial or early involvement of the distal airway, a site accessible only to droplets up to 5 μm in diameter.

The 4–6-hour cycle of replication is followed by viral release for several hours before cell death and progeny virions initiate infection in adjacent cells. Virus shedding occurs for 1–2 days before and about 5–7 days after the onset of symptoms and tends to be prolonged in young children and in immunocompromised patients.

The high infectivity of the virus, coupled with the short incubation period (about 2 days), high titres in nasopharyngeal secretions and the period of shedding, account for the rapid dissemination. In institutional settings, many individuals will be infected within 1–2 weeks. Influenza is an important cause of nosocomial infection and considerable morbidity and mortality can occur in acute medical wards, neonatal intensive care units and wards for the elderly.

Seasonality

Influenza demonstrates marked seasonality in many countries. This may be related to behavioural factors influencing exposure, including indoor crowding in bad weather, school activity and possibly the greater survival of virus in aerosols during the winter months.

Outbreaks often coincide with increased activity from respiratory syncytial virus and occur during periods when other respiratory pathogens, including coronaviruses, rhinoviruses and adenoviruses, are prevalent. Interpandemic epidemics of varying intensity occur virtually every year, almost exclusively during the winter months. Summertime outbreaks are reported occasionally in the northern hemisphere. Endemic year-long transmission is described in the tropics, with increased activity during wet seasons.

Outbreaks usually appear abruptly, peak within 2–3 weeks and tend to be of short duration (about 5–6 weeks). Nationwide epidemics may

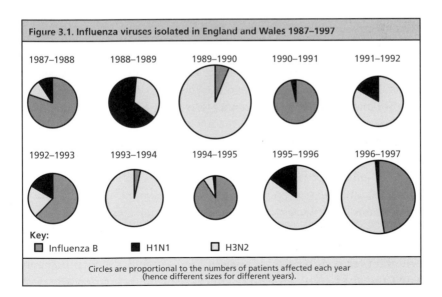

Figure 3.1. Influenza viruses isolated in England and Wales 1987–1997

| 1987–1988 | 1988–1989 | 1989–1990 | 1990–1991 | 1991–1992 |

| 1992–1993 | 1993–1994 | 1994–1995 | 1995–1996 | 1996–1997 |

Key:
☐ Influenza B   ■ H1N1   ☐ H3N2

Circles are proportional to the numbers of patients affected each year (hence different sizes for different years).

3

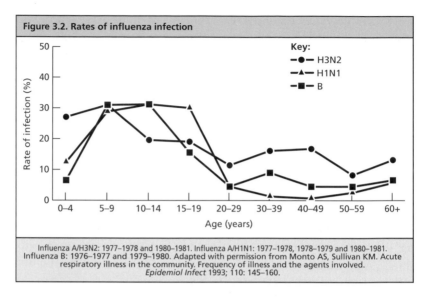

Figure 3.2. Rates of influenza infection

Key:
—●— H3N2
—▲— H1N1
—■— B

Influenza A/H3N2: 1977–1978 and 1980–1981. Influenza A/H1N1: 1977–1978, 1978–1979 and 1980–1981. Influenza B: 1976–1977 and 1979–1980. Adapted with permission from Monto AS, Sullivan KM. Acute respiratory illness in the community. Frequency of illness and the agents involved. *Epidemiol Infect* 1993; 110: 145–160.

last for about 3 months but successive or overlapping waves of infection by different subtypes of influenza A or by influenza A and B may result in a more prolonged outbreak.

Attack rates

Longitudinal studies in family and practice settings in the USA have provided valuable information on the annual occurrence of influenza, age-related attack rates, the ratio of subclinical to clinical infections and the difference in severity between A/H3N2 and A/H1N1 subtypes and influenza B. Many studies worldwide have identified that the highest attack rates occur in children and that school-aged children play a central role in the dissemination of influenza in households and the community. During epidemics, about 50% of households have one or more members who develop influenza virus infection and secondary attack rates among other family members average about 25%.

In a family study in Houston, USA, the risk of influenza during the first year of life was examined to provide information about the optimum time to initiate vaccination. One third of 209 infants monitored weekly for influenza were infected during their first year. Most infections occurred during the second 6 months of life; nine of 11 lower respiratory tract illnesses occurred in the older infants. The increase in maternal antibodies that should result from maternal immunization and the reduced risk of influenza in the early months suggest a time of about 6 months for active immunization of infants.

Mortality

Influenza epidemics are often accompanied by excess mortality (i.e. the difference between the number of deaths observed and the expected number in the absence of influenza). The burden of influenza on mortality is difficult to assess, however, because many deaths related to influenza are often attributed to other causes and seasonal factors such as ambient temperature and outbreaks of respiratory syncytial virus infection play a role.

In the UK, an estimated 5000–29 000 people died during each of the epidemics between 1975 and 1990; this is about 10 times the actual number of death certifications for influenza, indicating that influenza is responsible for many hidden deaths. In the USA, each of the 20 influenza seasons between 1972 and 1992 was associated with an average of 5600 pneumonia and influenza excess deaths (range 0–11 800) and 21 300 all-cause excess deaths (range 0–47 200). A/H3N2 seasons were associated with more deaths than A/H1N1 or influenza B seasons, corroborating clinical findings that the H3N2 virus is associated with greater morbidity. The cumulative mortality during recent interpandemic years is many-fold greater than the deaths associated with the three most recent pandemics.

Most influenza deaths occur in people aged at least 75 years. Whether age is an independent risk factor for influenza mortality is questionable because most deaths (about 84% during the 1989–1990 epidemic in England) occur in people with one or more underlying medical conditions. Patients identified as being at increased risk of death or hospitalization during epidemics or pandemics include those with chronic pulmonary disease (e.g. asthma, chronic bronchitis, emphysema, tuberculosis), rheumatic and ischaemic heart disease, diabetes mellitus, renal disease, neurological conditions (e.g. cerebrovascular disease, Parkinson's disease, multiple sclerosis) or anaemia and those who are pregnant or immunosuppressed (e.g. transplant recipients). The risk from influenza-related mortality increases with an increasing number of medical conditions suffered. It is also significantly higher among people living in residential care.

Nosocomial infections

Given the comparatively short incubation period of influenza, a patient with proven influenza or meeting an arbitrary clinical case definition can be designated as having a hospital-acquired infection if they had onset of illness after having been in a hospital or nursing home for 3 or more days.

Hospitals are complex dynamic environments in which patients, staff and visitors briefly intermingle. The extent of nosocomial influenza is uncertain and probably grossly underestimated because of the rapid turnover of patients and the infrequency of diagnostic testing. However, given the high attack rates of influenza (24–70%) during reported nosocomial outbreaks and given observations that about one in six winter cardiopulmonary admissions in the elderly and up to 20% of all paediatric admissions during a community outbreak have influenza, the opportunity for transmission from newly admitted patients appears high. Employees also represent an important route of virus entry into hospitals and long-term care facilities. During a comparatively mild epidemic season in Scotland in 1993–1994, serological evidence of influenza was found in 23% of 970 healthcare workers at four hospitals in Glasgow.

The morbidity and mortality from nosocomial influenza in the hospital setting is appreciable. Review of a number of reports indicates that more than one in 50 children and one in eight adults die from influenza acquired in hospital. Still higher mortality occurs in immunocompromised transplant recipients and those with haematological malignancy.

Outbreaks in nursing homes

Compared with elderly people in the community, nursing-home residents are at particular risk of serious influenza-related complications. They are older and have a higher rate of chronic ill health. Living in close proximity facilitates transmission and these patients may respond less readily to vaccination. Homes that experience influenza outbreaks (i.e. 10% of residents developing influenza-like illness within 1 week) tend to be larger (> 100 beds) and less well vaccinated (< 80% of residents immunized) than other establishments.

Influenza A subtypes H3N2 and H1N1 and influenza B have been co-circulating since 1977. All three types are usually detected each month globally but one virus normally predominates. Outbreaks with more than one influenza A subtype, with both influenza A and B or with both subtypes A/H3N2 and A/H1N1 and influenza B may occur during a single winter.

3

CHAPTER 4

Surveillance

- Influenza is subject to continuous, global surveillance, which is controlled by the WHO through regional and national centres
- Surveillance data are used to produce vaccines that are appropriate for the predominant circulating strains for the season and to give advanced warning of novel subtypes, especially those with pandemic potential

The WHO global surveillance system

Because of the variability of influenza viruses, the WHO in 1947 established an international network of laboratories to monitor the emergence and spread of new strains. The network's principal objectives are as follows.

- Early detection of novel subtypes of influenza A with pandemic potential
- Identification of antigenic variants to ensure continuing effectiveness of vaccines

The WHO collaborating centres maintain repositories of different virus strains, develop reagents and techniques for strain comparisons and train workers from national laboratories. They also have biocontainment facilities for the safe handling and investigation of viruses with pandemic potential.

National influenza laboratories perform virus isolations in egg or tissue culture and can identify virus isolates by haemagglutination inhibition (HAI) tests. Some also perform rapid viral diagnosis and titrate antibodies in human sera. They are provided with reagents for typing influenza isolates. Recent isolates are sent to the collaborating centres for comparison with one another, both antigenically and

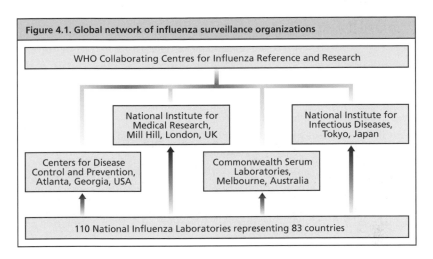

Figure 4.1. Global network of influenza surveillance organizations

4

genetically. In this way, the appearance and spread of new variants can be assessed.

This information enables recommendations to be made concerning the composition of influenza vaccine for use worldwide. These recommendations are made each year in February for the northern hemisphere and in September for the southern hemisphere.

In addition to the centres in Atlanta, London, Melbourne and Tokyo, the WHO has designated a collaborating centre in Memphis, Tennessee, USA, for the study of animal influenza viruses. This centre examines virus isolates from different animal species and the relationship between human and animal strains.

Regional surveillance systems

Regional surveillance systems such as the Pacific Basin Respiratory Virus Research Group and EUROGROG foster collaboration and exchange of information between different countries within a geographic region. EUROGROG is a network for the rapid exchange of epidemiological information between national influenza reference centres and other data-collecting institutions in Europe. The data are collected centrally in Paris, summarized, edited and redistributed to participating countries.

National surveillance

National influenza reference centres evaluate the activity of agents causing influenza-like illness, provide diagnostic facilities, obtain early virus isolations, identify the isolates and report to one of the four WHO collaborating centres. They may also collate information on the level of susceptibility of the local population by serological surveys. National surveillance centres also report the local influenza activity and warn of the onset and progression of seasonal epidemics.

The criteria for defining an epidemic vary from territory to territory. In England, for example, influenza is defined as epidemic according to consultation rates for 'influenza' and influenza-like illness. Rates of 50–200 per 100 000 consultations are usual when influenza viruses are circulating; rates exceeding 200 represent above-average influenza activity and rates above 400 are exceptional. Influenza activity may also be defined in terms of its effect on mortality: in the USA, if deaths attributable to pneumonia and influenza exceed 7.5% of total deaths, this is regarded as an influenza epidemic.

Many countries have a network of sentinel family doctors or primary care practitioners who notify the reference centres of cases of clinical influenza or influenza-like illness. Comparisons between illness rates must be interpreted with care; comparisons over time within a country are considered safe if the sample is sufficiently large and representative of the population as a whole. Schemes that incorporate virological surveillance are especially valuable but, even without these, weekly consultation rates usually correlate extremely well with laboratory reports of influenza and other non-specific indices, including pneumonia and influenza admissions and all-cause mortality.

Other sources or indices of clinical influenza activity include the following.

- Paediatricians
- The armed forces
- Sickness certification
- Sales of remedies for colds and influenza

- Private medical insurance claims
- Demand for emergency beds
- Hospital admissions for respiratory illness
- Mortality statistics

USA

Surveillance in the USA is carried out by state and territorial epidemiologists who notify weekly influenza activity. In addition about 140 family medical practitioners provide information on weekly consultation rates for influenza-like illness and some provide nasopharyngeal specimens to the Centers for Disease Control for virological assessment. The number of influenza virus isolations in around 70 laboratories is reported and mortality data from 122 cities are collected weekly. By providing mortality data within a few weeks, the impact of an epidemic may be seen during its evolution.

France

Two national reference centres, in Paris and Lyon, receive viruses obtained from hospitalized patients. Information on the occurrence of seven communicable diseases including influenza is provided by approximately 500 sentinel primary care practitioners (about 1% of French primary care practitioners). This allows the weekly national incidence per 100 000 population of influenza – defined as a febrile illness ($\geq 39°C$) with abrupt onset, myalgia and respiratory signs – to be calculated. In addition, weekly indices of influenza activity are provided by sales of non-prescription influenza-related drugs, the number of home visits by the emergency medical services, short-stay admissions, Social Security reports of short-term sickness (≤ 15 days) and deaths.

England, Wales and Scotland

The Public Health Laboratory Service Communicable Disease Surveillance Centre and Enteric and Respiratory Virus Laboratory monitor clinical and virological data for evidence of influenza activity. Surveillance schemes with sentinel primary care practitioners operate

31

in all three territories but each scheme uses different case definitions, so data cannot be compared directly. The Emergency Bed Service reports the number of emergency admissions to London hospitals. Weekly data on all-cause mortality in England and Wales and the numbers of deaths due to respiratory diseases are provided by the Office for National Statistics.

Virus isolations and other confirmatory results obtained in the Public Health Laboratory Service, National Health Service and some private laboratories are reported to the Communicable Disease Surveillance Centre weekly. The Enteric and Respiratory Virus Laboratory provides a reference facility for subtyping and genetic characterization of influenza isolates from hospital laboratories.

Germany

A German network of approximately 600 sentinel primary care physicians and paediatricians was set up in 1992. Data on the weekly numbers of acute respiratory infections in five age bands and the weekly number of consultations are transmitted to a central computer. Data on hospitalization, mortality and sick leave are collated and virological surveillance is provided through weekly collection of swabs in physicians' offices and hospitals.

Other countries

National surveillance schemes similar to the ones described above evaluate influenza virus activity in many countries in the Americas, Europe, Asia, Australasia, Oceania and Africa.

> Influenza has no pathognomonic clinical features, so the impact of the disease is quantified by virological surveillance and assessment of the contribution of influenza to illness and death in the community.

CHAPTER 5

The clinical picture

- Diagnosis can be made accurately in up to 70% of adults on clinical grounds alone
- Influenza in children is similar to adult infection, except that drowsiness occurs in up to 50% of cases; fever is also more prominent in children
- The major complications of influenza are respiratory and include bronchitis, croup, bronchiolitis, pneumonia (viral and bacterial), lung abscess, empyema and exacerbations of existing lung disease
- Influenza infection can lead to cardiovascular, neurological, psychiatric and other systemic illness: evidence from the 1957–1958 pandemic suggests that CNS complications (excluding febrile convulsions) are not uncommon and may include toxic encephalopathy, viral encephalitis, secondary bacterial meningitis and psychiatric events
- Influenza infection causes serious complications in immunosuppressed patients, including graft rejection and prolonged viral shedding
- Pregnant women with influenza appear to be at increased risk of hospitalization
- Renal failure, caused by myoglobinuria in influenza A infection is an infrequent complication, occurring most often in young adults

Introduction

Clinicians in various specialties can expect to see influenza in one or more of its guises each winter. It causes a broad spectrum of illness, ranging from asymptomatic infection to pneumonia and multisystem complications. The clinical course is affected by the inherent properties of the virus, by the patient's age, immune status, smoking, comorbidities (e.g. chronic heart and lung diseases), renal failure and immunosuppression and by pregnancy.

Uncomplicated influenza in adults

The onset of symptoms is typically abrupt, with prominent systemic features including malaise, feverishness, chills, headache, anorexia, myalgia and dizziness. Fever of 38–40°C is the most prominent sign of infection; pyrexia peaks at the height of systemic features and may last for 1–5 days. Early symptoms include a non-productive cough, nasal discharge, sneezing and sore throat; less frequently, patients may have productive cough, hoarseness and substernal soreness. Crackles and wheezing are heard in about 10% of patients. These symptoms and signs last for 3–5 days, although cough, lassitude and malaise may persist for 1–2 weeks after the fever subsides.

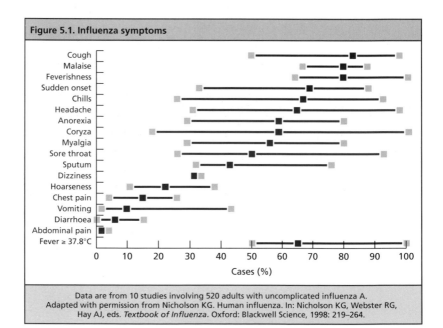

Figure 5.1. Influenza symptoms

Cases (%)

Data are from 10 studies involving 520 adults with uncomplicated influenza A.
Adapted with permission from Nicholson KG. Human influenza. In: Nicholson KG, Webster RG, Hay AJ, eds. *Textbook of Influenza*. Oxford: Blackwell Science, 1998: 219–264.

Comparative studies suggest that A/H3N2 infections produce more severe illness than A/H1N1 and influenza B is intermediate in severity. Illnesses tend to be more severe during the first and second waves of pandemics because of lack of immunity. Gastrointestinal symptoms may be more prominent in the elderly.

Diagnosing adult influenza

Influenza is associated with a range of clinical syndromes that can be caused by other respiratory viruses. Cough and fever are the most valuable symptoms in characterizing influenza A and B. Recent trials of NA inhibitors have shown that, when local surveillance detects the presence of influenza in the community, the likelihood of diagnosing influenza clinically is around 60–70% (mean of five studies, using the criteria in Figure 5.2, 2154/3466 patients or 62%).

The success in diagnosing influenza in treatment studies using the above clinical criteria does not reflect the recent experience of primary care physicians in Europe and North America. For example, in a study of 361 patients in England during the winters of 1992–1993 and 1993–1994, only 35% of children aged 0–4 years and 22% of adults aged over 65 years with an influenza-like illness had virologically confirmed influenza. Collectively, the data tell us that doctors can substantially

Figure 5.2. Criteria for influenza diagnosis: NA inhibitor trials	
Zanamivir trials	**GS 4104 trials**
Fever (≥ 37.8°C) and/or feverishness	Fever (≥ 38°C)
plus	plus
TWO of:	ONE of:
Cough Sore throat Myalgia Headache	Cough Sore throat Nasal symptoms
	plus
	ONE of:
	Feverishness Malaise Headache Myalgia or prostration

improve their diagnosis of influenza by using the diagnostic criteria in Figure 5.2 when influenza is known to be circulating locally.

Influenza in children

Although the manifestations of influenza in children are similar to those in adults – sudden onset with fever, headache, cough and sore throat – some age-related differences are apparent. Drowsiness (uncommon in adults) occurs in about 50% of children less than 4 years old but in only 10% of children aged 5–14 years. Gastrointestinal symptoms (e.g. nausea, vomiting, central abdominal pain, diarrhoea) occur in up to 40% of children. Otitis media complicates about 25% of infections in young seronegative children and occurred during 67% of influenza A infections in otitis-prone 1–3-year-old children. Fever also tends to be more prominent in children, whereas myalgia, sweats, sputum production and other respiratory symptoms are more common in adults.

Infants beyond the age when maternally derived antibodies provide protection and those with congenital abnormalities are at increased risk from the complications of influenza.

Hospitalizations and deaths

Between 0.5% and 1% of influenza infections in children aged less than 5 years result in hospitalization. During the peak epidemic months of 13 consecutive influenza A epidemics and six influenza B epidemics, influenza accounted for 36% and 11% of all hospitalizations for respiratory illness in children under 8 years old. The impact of influenza on paediatric hospitalization is undoubtedly underestimated because the disease often manifests with non-respiratory complications.

Figure 5.3. Respiratory complication rates in hospitalized children during influenza A outbreaks	
Complication	Children affected (%)
Acute bronchitis	12 – 26
Croup	5 – 15
Radiographic evidence of pneumonia	5 – 8

One infant in 5000 in the community dies during epidemics of influenza A and B.

Complications of paediatric influenza infection

- **Exacerbation of asthma:** in Nigeria, influenza A infection was found in 16% of 74 children hospitalized with asthmatic exacerbations. About 75% of asthmatic children with influenza suffer an exacerbation. Investigators have observed declines in forced expiratory volume in 1 second of up to 75%
- **Exacerbation of cystic fibrosis:** influenza has been implicated in 4–13% of cases
- **Febrile convulsions** in 20–50% of children hospitalized with influenza
- **Abdominal pain:** among hospital admissions, there may be a predominance of gastrointestinal manifestations – abdominal pain, diarrhoea, vomiting – that mimic appendicitis
- **Myalgia** affecting the legs and back occurs early on, whereas **myositis** (and **myoglobinuria** with or without renal failure) is an infrequent complication generally occurring during the recovery phase. Myositis mostly occurs with influenza B; typically, leg pain and muscle tenderness last 1–5 days
- **Reye's syndrome:** probably because of reduced salicylate use, recent trends in the USA and UK indicate a decreased incidence of influenza-related Reye's syndrome

5

Influenza in the elderly

Influenza in the elderly is associated with a higher incidence of lower respiratory tract symptoms of sputum production, wheeze or chest pain than in young adults or children. About half of elderly patients with symptomatic virologically confirmed influenza consult their medical practitioner.

Between one in 250 and one in 100 people over 65 years old in a health-maintenance organization in Minnesota, USA, were admitted to hospital for 'pneumonia and influenza' during each of the six influenza seasons from 1990 to 1996. The observation that vaccination was associated with an overall reduction of 39% for these admissions suggests that a substantial number are influenza-related.

During the same study, one in 250 to one in 50 elderly people were hospitalized each winter with heart failure. Vaccination was associated with an overall reduction of 27% for congestive heart failure admissions, suggesting that many are influenza-related. In Rochester, New York, USA, 16% of 210 patients admitted with virologically confirmed influenza A had a discharge diagnosis of congestive heart failure. This shows that a substantial number of influenza admissions in the elderly develop cardiovascular complications and that many are hidden as heart failure.

5

Respiratory complications

The complications of influenza are predominantly respiratory and include acute bronchitis, laryngotracheobronchitis (croup), bronchiolitis, pneumonia, lung abscess, empyema, exacerbations of chronic bronchitis, asthma and cystic fibrosis, pneumothorax and surgical emphysema.

Acute bronchitis

Acute bronchitis is the most common lower respiratory tract complication of influenza, occurring in up to 30% of patients. It manifests as a dry, harsh cough that is often more severe at night and may progress to become productive. It occurs more frequently with increasing age and chronic medical conditions.

Pneumonia

Pneumonia has been identified in 5–38% of patients with influenza A and in up to 10% of patients with influenza B. Two main types of pneumonia are recognized: a primary viral pneumonia and a secondary bacterial pneumonia (the latter occurring either with viral pneumonia or as a late complication). During the 1957–1958 pandemic, around 25% of fatal pneumonias were viral and the lungs of most patients with secondary bacterial pneumonia were co-infected with influenza.

Patients with pneumonia can deteriorate rapidly. During the 1989–1990 epidemic in Leicestershire, UK, 78 of 156 patients admitted to hospital with pneumonia and influenza died during hospitalization. More than one third succumbed within 48 hours and fewer than one third survived for longer than 8 days.

Primary influenzal pneumonia

Patients present with a typical onset of influenza followed abruptly by increasing cough, chest pain and dyspnoea. The interval between onset of illness and pneumonia is typically 2–3 days. Auscultation reveals crackles or wheezes, or both, but no signs of consolidation. Poor outcome is heralded by profound dyspnoea, tachypnoea, cyanosis and haemoptysis and, terminally, by shock and signs of pulmonary oedema. Death occurs within 4–5 days of onset.

5

Secondary bacterial pneumonia

Almost three quarters of patients with fatal or life-threatening influenzal pneumonia have a secondary bacterial infection. *Staphylococcus aureus*, either as sole pathogen or with other micro-organisms, was identified in most cases during the 1957–1958 pandemic and was also prominent in the 1968–1970 pandemic.

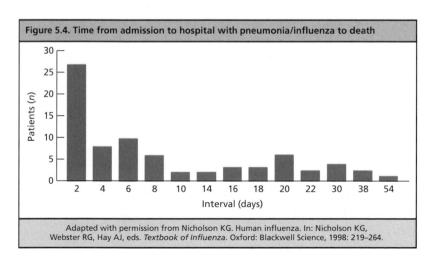

Figure 5.4. Time from admission to hospital with pneumonia/influenza to death

Adapted with permission from Nicholson KG. Human influenza. In: Nicholson KG, Webster RG, Hay AJ, eds. *Textbook of Influenza*. Oxford: Blackwell Science, 1998: 219–264.

In about one third of cases, increasing respiratory symptoms are continuous with influenzal symptoms. Alternatively, a brief improvement of influenzal symptoms is followed, 4–5 days after onset (or occasionally several weeks later), by recrudescence of fever, cough productive of purulent sputum and worsening dyspnoea. Examination often reveals areas of consolidation affecting one or more lobes, diffuse crackles and wheezing.

The mortality from staphylococcal pneumonia – around 28% during the 1957–1958 pandemic – was more than twice as high as from other influenzal pneumonias (12%). It was similar in all age groups and in those with and without underlying high-risk conditions, whereas mortality from other influenza-associated pneumonias was concentrated in those with chronic medical conditions and in people aged at least 55 years.

Up to 50% of patients with staphylococcal pneumonia and 35% of those with other forms of pneumonia during pandemics have no underlying medical conditions. This states the case for much wider use of vaccines when a new pandemic strain emerges.

Other respiratory complications

- **Exacerbation of asthma:** severe epidemics of influenza result in a small but significant excess mortality attributed to asthma
- **Exacerbation of chronic obstructive airways disease:** up to 28% of exacerbations are associated with influenza A or B
- **Exacerbation of cystic fibrosis:** acute upper respiratory viral infection is associated with exacerbations of cystic fibrosis, secondary bacterial infection and disease progression
- **Lung abscess:** radiography does not reflect the true incidence of abscess formation during the acute stages of bacterial pneumonia. Frank abscess formation was found *post mortem* in around one in six people during the 1957–1958 pandemic
- **Empyema:** found in 10–20% of fatal cases during the 1918–1920 pandemic but in only 1% of patients with pneumonia during the pandemic of Asian influenza in 1957–1958
- **Invasive pulmonary aspergillosis:** reported on at least eight occasions as a complication of influenza A in immunocompetent patients

Other manifestations

Toxic shock syndrome

Toxic shock syndrome is an unusual complication of influenza with secondary staphylococcal infection. By 1993, a total of 15 cases had been described, 12 as a complication of influenza B; overall mortality was 40%.

Intensive care

Little information is available on admissions to intensive care units for influenza. Such patients represent a potential source of nosocomial spread of infection to the highly vulnerable. Occasionally, patients with influenza may be admitted with pneumonia or additional life-threatening complications, such as the following.

- **Reye's syndrome:** seen primarily in children (peak onset 5–14 years); histologically confirmed cases have occurred in adults
- **Encephalopathy, encephalitis** and **Guillain–Barré syndrome**
- **Toxic shock syndrome**

Cardiac involvement

Electrocardiographic abnormalities have been found in up to 81% of patients with influenza in hospital and in 43% of patients in the community, mostly in people without cardiac symptoms. These abnormalities may be transient, lasting no longer than 24 hours, but occasionally persist for months or years and the underlying disorders may cause fatal arrhythmias or restrictive cardiomyopathy long after recovery from influenza. Myocarditis, common in influenza, is mostly asymptomatic.

Diabetes mellitus

People with Type II (non-insulin-dependent) diabetes mellitus are 1.7 times more likely to die from pneumonia and influenza than the general population. In one study, six of nine diabetic patients with influenzal pneumonia died.

During epidemics of influenza A in 1968–1970 and 1972–1973, pneumonia and influenza deaths increased more than fourfold from 104 per 100 000 in people with chronic cardiovascular disease to 481 per 100 000 (i.e. one in 208) in patients with both cardiovascular disease and diabetes. Deaths from diabetes increased by 5–12% during six of seven epidemics between 1957 and 1966.

Studies of the effectiveness of influenza vaccine in preventing hospital admissions in people with diabetes provide insight into the impact of influenza in this population. During epidemics in 1989–1990 and 1993 in Leicestershire, UK, the estimated effectiveness of influenza vaccine in reducing hospital admissions was 79%, suggesting that a substantial proportion of admissions during epidemics among people with diabetes are related to influenza.

Neurological disorders

Although dementia, seizure disorders, cerebrovascular disease, difficulty with oropharyngeal secretions and neuromuscular disease have all been identified as risk factors for the development of pneumonia, the evidence that chronic CNS disorders increase the risk from influenza is not strong. People with Parkinson's disease are three to four times more likely to die from pneumonia and influenza than the general population, presumably because of their relative immobility in the later stages. During the 1989–1990 epidemic, chronic neurological disease emerged as a risk factor for influenzal death but not for hospitalization.

CNS complications

Reports from the 1957–1958 pandemic suggest that neurological complications, excluding febrile convulsions in children, are not uncommon. In patients with neurological complications associated with influenza A/H1N1 and A/H3N2 and influenza B, convulsions represent the most common CNS complication, affecting approximately one fifth of young children hospitalized with influenza.

The pyrexia, hypoxia and pH abnormalities that accompany influenza may be responsible for a toxic encephalopathy in some patients, whereas others develop viral encephalitis, an immune-mediated para-infectious encephalomyelitis or Reye's syndrome. Most patients recover fully, often shortly after the onset of influenza. However, the 1995 influenza epidemic in Japan was exceptionally neurovirulent and lethal.

Bacterial meningitis

An increase in meningococcal infection after the 1989–1990 influenza outbreak led UK investigators to undertake a case–control study. Patients with meningococcal disease were almost four times more likely than control patients to have been infected recently with influenza A. However, the proportion of meningococcal disease causally linked to influenza is small.

Cerebrovascular disease

A possible causal link between influenza and subarachnoid haemorrhage was suggested in 1978 by the finding of a fourfold increased incidence of antibodies to influenza A virus from patients with subarachnoid haemorrhage, compared with a neurological control group and age- and sex-matched patients.

Encephalitis lethargica

The global pandemic of encephalitis lethargica followed by post-encephalitic Parkinson's disease was claimed to be causally associated with the 1918–1920 influenza pandemic. Investigators have examined the possible association but the link remains unproven.

Psychiatric sequelae

Acute psychoses, some with auditory and visual hallucinations, developing 2–10 days after influenza in the pandemic of 1957–1958 were reported. These episodes may represent manifestations of encephalitis or immune-mediated para-infectious encephalitis.

Obstetric considerations

Pregnant women

Pregnant women appear to be at increased risk of severe pulmonary complications of influenza, with the possibility of hospitalization and death during the second and third trimesters. However, the absolute risk is small, particularly during interpandemic years. Analysis of mortality statistics in the UK during the 1989–1990 epidemic revealed a fourfold increase in deaths among pregnant women and showed that the epidemic accounted for about 90 excess deaths during pregnancy out of an estimated 25 185 total excess deaths.

Influenza complicating mitral-valve disease in pregnancy is associated with an overall mortality of around 45%, or higher (60%) if labour occurs during influenza. Few pregnant women hospitalized with influenza have high-risk chronic medical conditions. To minimize the risks, all pregnant women would need to be immunized.

Unborn children

Concern has been expressed in three main areas, as follows.

- **Congenital abnormalities:** although an increase in various congenital abnormalities after influenzal illness during pregnancy has been reported, no consistent association between specific defects and illness has been found and the virus has not been conclusively implicated
- **Childhood leukaemia:** some studies have shown a possible relationship between maternal influenza and childhood leukaemia. This is not a constant finding and the effect, if real, is considered to be very small
- **Schizophrenia:** studies have yielded conflicting results. Even if a real association between prenatal exposure to influenza and development of schizophrenia exists, the relationship is not necessarily causal because influenza may lead to drug therapy for symptom relief and obstetric complications (the latter having been reported in association with the later development of schizophrenia)

The available data do not imply that maternal influenza should be an indication for termination of pregnancy.

Stillbirths, perinatal and neonatal mortality

In early 1986, a small cluster of early and late fetal deaths prompted a study that revealed that case pregnancies had a significant excess of recent influenza-like illness and were significantly more likely than controls to have serological evidence of influenza A infection.

Review of mortality statistics in England and Wales in 1921–1932 revealed a 7–12% increase in deaths from premature births during months with the highest influenza death rates. Neonatal mortality in England and Wales in the second quarter of 1970, after a major influenza epidemic, increased by 9%. Similar increases of infant mortality occurred in relation to four of five other major influenza epidemics (1951, 1953, 1959 and 1961); the exception was the Asian influenza pandemic of 1957–1958.

Perinatal deaths in England and Wales increased 1.6-fold during the 1989–1990 epidemic. The data suggest that, for around every 3000 births in a 12-month period, one perinatal death occurred during the epidemic.

Immunosuppression

Patients up to 19 years of age with any form of cancer who are receiving immunosuppressive therapy or who have received such treatment during the preceding year have a significantly higher incidence of symptomatic influenza infection (32%) than community controls (14%).

Immunosuppressed patients are more susceptible to influenza and are at higher risk of developing pneumonia and dying. Most fatal pneumonias complicating influenza in immunocompromised patients are viral.

Graft rejection

In transplant recipients, influenza A and B infection may lead to graft rejection and loss, possibly due to interruption of chemotherapy. Allograft rejection occurred in four of 12 paediatric solid organ transplant recipients infected with influenza B.

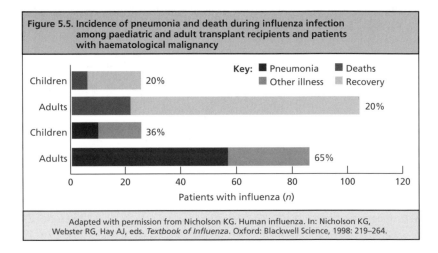

Figure 5.5. Incidence of pneumonia and death during influenza infection among paediatric and adult transplant recipients and patients with haematological malignancy

Adapted with permission from Nicholson KG. Human influenza. In: Nicholson KG, Webster RG, Hay AJ, eds. *Textbook of Influenza*. Oxford: Blackwell Science, 1998: 219–264.

Prolonged virus shedding

Almost 70% of influenza A or B infections diagnosed in immunocompromised patients in hospital are nosocomial. Immunosuppressed patients with influenza can shed influenza virus for up to 5 months. Viruses from such patients can develop resistance to amantadine and rimantadine rapidly and pose a significant threat to other patients.

HIV

Little evidence of an increase in morbidity or mortality from influenza in patients infected with HIV has been found, although prolonged febrile illness has been described. Shedding of influenza virus may be prolonged in children infected with HIV.

In cities with a high incidence of HIV infection, an increase in pneumonia deaths among people aged 25–44 years during the peak influenza months provides the only other evidence supporting an increase in severity of influenza in adults with HIV.

Renal failure

Rhabdomyolysis, with myoglobinaemia, myoglobinuria and acute renal failure is reported in association with influenza, usually in young adults with influenza A. During outbreaks, influenza A is probably the leading cause of acute myoglobinuric renal failure.

Haemorrhage and disseminated intravascular coagulation

Bleeding disorders in influenza may be due in part to disseminated intravascular coagulation, which has been associated with both influenza A and B. Patients may present with haemoptysis, haematuria, haematemesis, malaena, vaginal bleeding, purpura, renal failure and jaundice.

Haemophagocytic syndrome and aplastic anaemia

Virus-associated haemophagocytic syndrome, which occurs mostly in association with cytomegalovirus and Epstein–Barr virus, has been linked with influenza. It tends to resolve within several months. Aplastic anaemia has also been linked with influenza A.

5

Recognition of influenza by doctors, nurses and patients is increasingly important, so that treatment and prophylaxis can be started to control infection both in the community and in high-risk settings.

CHAPTER 6

Diagnosis

- Diagnosis and identification of influenza serve three main purposes: to allow surveillance of influenza activity, to assist in tailoring therapy to disease and to produce vaccines
- Specimens for analysis are either respiratory tract swabs, washes or aspirates (containing the virus or its antigens) or blood samples that confirm diagnosis by the presence of antibodies
- Diagnosis may become more important as new therapeutic options become more widely available

Introduction

Laboratory identification of prevailing strains is essential for epidemiological purposes and vaccine production. However, in terms of clinical management, current methods of diagnosis do not lend themselves to providing results that could influence the initiation of treatment. Influenza is diagnosed clinically correctly in around 60–70% of patients with a characteristic febrile illness when a local outbreak is virologically confirmed. The availability of sensitive, specific and more rapid (point-of-care) diagnostic tests could help to ensure that outbreaks of respiratory illness are confirmed quickly as influenza, thereby giving confidence in the level of accuracy of clinical diagnosis. Rapid diagnosis of influenza is also important to control infection in high-risk settings.

Collection and transport of specimens

Human influenza viruses replicate in the respiratory tract epithelium and are transmitted through the release of infectious particles into respiratory secretions. Two types of specimen are collected to confirm the diagnosis: respiratory tract specimens (to identify the virus, viral antigens or nucleic acid) and acute and convalescent blood samples (to confirm the diagnosis serologically).

Specimens of choice

The diagnostic yield is improved by the collection of clinical specimens containing virally infected epithelial cells as early in the course of illness as possible, preferably within the first 3 days. Nasopharyngeal washes and aspirates contain more cellular material than nasopharyngeal swabs and, providing a better yield of virus, these are the specimens of choice. Throat swabs or gargles are of less value. Sputum alone should not be collected in preference to other respiratory specimens.

Nose swabs

6

Nose swabs are obtained with a dry cotton-, rayon- or dacron-tipped swab. Swabs with wooden shafts should be avoided because preservatives used in their manufacture may leak out and affect the cells. Similarly, calcium alginate swabs should not be used because the alginate can also inhibit cultures.

Nose swabs should not be collected from the anterior nares. Instead, the swab is inserted through the nares until resistance is met at the level of the turbinate, then rotated vigorously around the entire surface; the process is repeated on the opposite side. The tips of the swabs are cut or broken off into screw-capped vials containing viral transport medium. Alternatively, the swabs can be agitated in the viral transport medium; the fluid is expressed from the tip and the swab is removed.

Nasopharyngeal aspirates

Specimens from the nasopharynx can be obtained by aspirating secretions collected from beyond the anterior nares with a fine-bore catheter connected to a mucus extractor. The specimens should be collected from the posterior pharyngeal wall, which is lined with respiratory epithelium. The catheter should therefore be thin enough to reach as far as the posterior pharyngeal wall (French gauge 8 for infants and small children, 12 for adults) and should be rounded to avoid trauma.

Both nasal passages should be sampled. Suction is applied either by ward suction or by a portable suction machine; alternatively, aspiration may be carried out using a 20 ml syringe. A small volume of viral transport medium or saline solution is sucked through the catheter after its removal from the nose to wash any residual mucus and cellular material into the trap.

Nasal washes

Nasal washes are obtained by instilling 3–5 ml sterile phosphate-buffered saline solution or viral transport medium into each nostril with the head angled backwards. The patient is instructed to close the upper airway (Valsalva manoeuvre) and not to swallow. Fluid is collected in a sterile container by tilting the head forwards and blowing through the nose. Alternatively, approximately 2 ml sterile phosphate-buffered saline solution or viral transport medium can be inoculated into the nose, using fine-bore tubing or a catheter attached to a 5 ml syringe and immediately aspirated back into the syringe. Saline phosphate-buffered washes are placed into an equal volume of viral transport medium.

Severely ill patients and fatal cases

Endotracheal and bronchoalveolar lavage fluid may be useful for detection of influenza infections of the lung and lower airways. Warmed saline solution or viral transport medium (50–60 ml) is introduced though the bronchoscope into the affected portion of the lung and removed by suction into suitable containers.

Virus recovery may be attempted from the heart in patients with myocarditis and from muscle in patients with Reye's syndrome or myositis. Post-mortem specimens should be obtained as soon after death as possible.

Transport

Specimens for virus isolation should be transported in viral transport medium on wet ice and maintained at 4°C before inoculation or

6

immunofluorescence. The isolation rate is effectively unchanged when specimens are held at 4°C for up to 4 days. Virus has also been recovered for up to 5 days after collection from samples sent by post.

Virus isolation

Influenza viruses can be isolated in 10–11-day-old embryonated hens' eggs and in various primary, diploid and continuous cell cultures. Influenza virus is one of only a few human pathogens that grow in eggs and produce haemagglutination activity. The whole process of identifying a culture-positive sample as influenza virus takes about 4–5 days. Rapid culture assays, which detect viruses in cultured cells by immunological techniques, take about 1–3 days and have a sensitivity of 56–100% in comparison with standard culture.

6

Subtyping of virus isolates

Differentiation of influenza A and B viruses and of the subtypes of influenza A is usually carried out by HAI tests using panels of specific antisera. Alternatively, detection of viral nucleic acid by reverse transcriptase polymerase chain reaction (PCR) can be used to distinguish between types and subtypes of influenza.

Antigen detection

Immunofluorescence

Viral antigen can be detected in respiratory secretions by direct fluorescent or indirect antibody staining of exfoliated nasal epithelial cells. The sensitivity of immunofluorescence in comparison with culture is around 50–90%. Immunofluorescence is labour intensive and requires a high degree of technical expertise, in contrast to other, more rapid antigen detection systems.

Immunoassays

Influenzal antigen is detected in respiratory secretions by various immunological techniques, including enzyme, membrane, radio-, optical and fluoro-immunoassays. These assays can be applied directly to clinical specimens, cell-culture supernatants or cell lysates. They commonly depend on the capture of viral nucleoprotein and its interaction with monoclonal antibodies. Generally, such tests give 50–80% sensitivity in comparison with virus isolation.

Self-contained rapid diagnostic kits

Tests such as the Directigen^{TM} Flu A test, which can take less than 15 minutes to complete, can make important contributions to individual case management and control of influenza A infection. The Directigen^{TM} Flu A kit, for relatively simple identification of influenza A only, uses a nasopharyngeal specimen, which is assayed for influenza A antigens using a membrane immunosorbent method. Although it is more simple and rapid than conventional enzyme-linked immunosorbent assay techniques, the process is still probably too labour intensive for use in primary care practices, especially during the busy influenza season. Newer tests that can distinguish between influenza A and B are currently being evaluated.

Viral RNA detection

Reverse transcriptase PCR can be used to type and subtype influenza infections using clinical specimens or virus grown in cell culture or eggs. PCR can detect and quantify the presence of viral RNA of influenza virus A and B, human para-influenza virus types 1, 2 and 3 and respiratory syncytial viruses A and B in nasal specimens in a single test. Tests have demonstrated 100% sensitivity and 98% specificity. PCR may be more sensitive than culture and the technique can detect influenza viruses harbouring mutations associated with antiviral resistance. However, PCR is labour intensive and more expensive and slower (1–2 days) than antigen detection tests.

Serology

Serological tests are of little practical value in patient management. Although immunoglobulin (Ig) M antibodies can be detected in almost

90% of patients with influenza A, a serum IgM antibody response is detected on admission in only about one third of patients. Thus, an IgM antibody response is less sensitive than antigen detection in confirming influenza early during the illness.

The demonstration of a fourfold or greater rise in antibody titre when acute and convalescent sera are compared is indicative of infection.

Complement fixation test

The complement fixation test is relatively insensitive but it has the advantage of being unaffected by non-specific inhibitors and, because it measures antibodies to the influenza nucleoprotein, which is conserved, it can be used to detect antibody rises to new antigenic variants.

Haemagglutination inhibition test

The HAI test is based on the property of influenza viruses to agglutinate erythrocytes and of antibodies to the HA to interfere with this process. It is a comparatively straightforward test, requiring no complex or expensive equipment, but suffers the disadvantage that pretreatment of sera is required to prevent false-positive reactions. Fourfold or greater rises in HAI antibodies occur in 70–90% of infections. HAI assays are routinely used to assess the immune response to vaccination. HAI antibody is subtype- and strain-specific and this property can be used to demonstrate antigenic drift.

Enzyme immunoassays

Significantly more infections with influenza virus are detected by enzyme immunoassays than by complement fixation test and HAI tests. Enzyme immunoassays also provide the means to measure IgG, IgA and IgM antibody subclasses secreted in respiratory secretions. However, subtype specificity is not observed and no close association is found between measures of IgG and protection. These observations suggest that, although enzyme immunoassays show greater diagnostic efficacy than other tests, HAI remains the serological method of choice in determining the subtype causing infection and the immune status.

6

Figure 6.1. Haemagglutination inhibition testing of sera

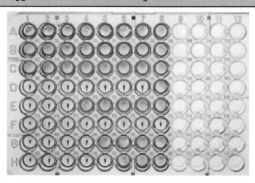

Reproduced with permission from Zambon M. Laboratory diagnosis of influenza. In: Nicholson KG, Webster RG, Hay AJ, eds. *Textbook of Influenza*. Oxford: Blackwell Science, 1998: 291–313.

6

Neutralization tests

Neutralization tests can be carried out in eggs or in tissue culture. They are more complex than the HAI test, require a greater level of expertise and take several days to complete.

Improved diagnostic techniques, enabling rapid virological confirmation of influenza infection, will have benefits in patient management and infection control. Early diagnosis will become increasingly important as novel, specific treatments for influenza, such as the NA inhibitors, become available.

CHAPTER 7

Vaccination and infection control

- Vaccines are rated according to their efficacy (precise, influenza-specific outcomes) and effectiveness (clinically relevant but non-specific 'real-world' outcomes, such as number of hospitalizations)
- Vaccines can be manufactured from inactivated virus, split virions, purified surface antigens and live-attenuated influenza virus
- Vaccine strains have to be selected annually from those circulating in the population, in an attempt to prevent those strains from infecting at-risk groups
- Recommendations for vaccination vary from country to country but commonly include the elderly, cardiopulmonary patients, patients with metabolic disorders (especially diabetes), the immunocompromised, nursing-home residents and healthcare workers

7

Vaccine efficacy

Vaccine efficacy is calculated by comparing the rate of virologically confirmed illness in vaccinees with the rate in non-vaccinated controls. Because the annual attack rate of symptomatic influenza in an adult population is usually no higher than 5–10% and the proportion who develop pneumonia may be of a similar magnitude, studies of vaccine efficacy need to be extremely large to detect a real difference in outcomes in the two groups. Most vaccines in clinical practice have efficacies greater than 70%.

Clinical effectiveness

Clinical effectiveness is determined by the observed reduction in clinically relevant but non-specific outcomes, such as influenza-like

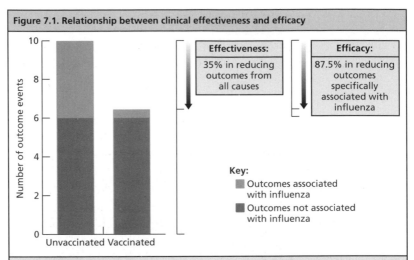

Figure 7.1. Relationship between clinical effectiveness and efficacy

Number of outcome events (y-axis: 0, 2, 4, 6, 8, 10)

Unvaccinated Vaccinated

Effectiveness: 35% in reducing outcomes from all causes

Efficacy: 87.5% in reducing outcomes specifically associated with influenza

Key:
Outcomes associated with influenza
Outcomes not associated with influenza

In this hypothetical example, influenza vaccination was associated with a 35% reduction in all outcomes, although only 40% of outcomes were complications of influenza. Thus, the underlying efficacy of the vaccine for preventing influenza-associated outcomes would be 87.5% (35% ÷ 40%). Adapted with permission from Nichol KL. Efficacy/clinical effectiveness of inactivated influenza virus vaccines in adults. In: Nicholson KG, Webster RG, Hay AJ, eds. *Textbook of Influenza*. Oxford: Blackwell Science, 1998: 358–372.

illness, hospitalizations for pneumonia or deaths from all causes. Vaccine effectiveness is measured by comparing the rates of illness in vaccinees and non-vaccinees and estimates of vaccine effectiveness are generally considerably lower than vaccine efficacy.

Inactivated vaccines

After the first isolation of human influenza virus in 1933, early breakthroughs in vaccine development came with the demonstration in 1937 that influenza virus could be grown in hens' eggs and then with the recognition that influenza causes haemagglutination. The development of the haemagglutination test enabled the potency of vaccines to be measured and the HAI test also provided the means to titrate large numbers of sera for antibodies to the virus.

During controlled trials conducted in many thousands of military recruits in the US Army over several decades, vaccine efficacy for reducing laboratory-confirmed influenza was 80–90% during seven of 14 seasons, around 70% during five and less than 40% during only two seasons.

Strategies for vaccination against influenza

- **Whole-virion vaccine:** although whole-virion vaccines are more pure than they used to be, they are considered unsuitable for use in young children
- **Split-virus vaccine:** numerous trials have shown that split-virus vaccines, now the most common type of influenza vaccine, are as immunogenic as whole-virion material in primed patients but less reactogenic, particularly in children. However, they are not as immunogenic as whole-virion vaccines in vaccine-naive patients during antigenic shift or in young children who have not been previously infected, in which case, a second dose of vaccine is required
- **Surface-antigen vaccine:** these contain purified HA and NA and are as immunogenic as whole-virion and split-virus vaccines in primed patients, although two doses are required in young children
- **High-growth reassortants:** newly isolated influenza viruses often grow poorly in hens' eggs. Because low virus yields limit the amount of material for vaccine production, producing sufficient vaccine using such strains would be difficult and expensive. To overcome this problem, genetic reassortants are produced between new isolates and a virus with excellent growth characteristics

7

Potential future developments

- **Adjuvants:** these are under evaluation to enhance the immune response to vaccination. So far only one, aluminium hydroxide, has been licensed for use in humans but no benefit has been seen in clinical trials
- **Cell-culture vaccines**
- **Mucosal delivery**

Limitations of current vaccine manufacture

- Current influenza vaccines are produced in embryonated hens' eggs. Because of the large numbers required, advanced planning must commence nearly 1 year before vaccination
- Chickens are susceptible to disease, so an adequate supply of eggs and vaccine cannot be guaranteed
- In the event of a pandemic, vaccine production is unlikely to match global needs
- The interval between identification of a new pandemic strain and outbreaks may be insufficient to produce vaccine using current technology
- Growth of human influenza virus in eggs can lead to the selection of variants that differ antigenically from the original
- The requirement for high-growth reassortants can delay vaccine manufacture and reassortants may be unstable

7

Cell cultures as substrates for production of vaccine

The WHO has recognized an urgent need to develop a cell-culture technique for influenza vaccine production. Cell-culture systems offer the following advantages.

- Viruses isolated and passaged exclusively in mammalian cells retain their antigenic characteristics
- Virus growth occurs adequately in mammalian cells without the need for high-growth reassortants
- Vaccine production can be increased at short notice to meet unexpected demand or supplemental vaccine can be produced if a new variant is detected

Two continuous cell lines, Madin–Darby canine kidney (MDCK) cells and African green monkey kidney (Vero) cells, support influenza virus replication at levels sufficient to be considered for vaccine production. Candidate vaccines produced using both techniques are currently being evaluated. Vero cells are used currently to manufacture polio vaccine. The use of MDCK cells as a cell substrate for vaccine manufacture is under consideration.

Mucosal delivery

The need to give inactivated vaccines by injection represents a barrier to annual immunization. Interest has therefore been focused on alternative delivery systems, including mucosal administration by the intranasal or oral routes, which could prove more acceptable, cause fewer reactions and stimulate mucosal and humoral immunity.

Cold-adapted intranasal vaccine

A live, cold-adapted intranasal virus vaccine (FluMist™) is in the advanced stages of development and has undergone extensive clinical evaluation in adults and children. The vaccine is likely to be available soon.

In addition to the easy route of administration, the key advantage of administering influenza vaccine intranasally is that mucosal immunity (in the form of secretory antibodies) is induced, providing the strongest possible front line against influenza infection. The vaccine uses a live-attenuated (i.e. cold-adapted) strain, containing the genes for HA and NA antigens from the currently circulating influenza strains. By using a cold-adapted virus, viral replication occurs only at the lower temperatures of the nasopharynx and growth is inhibited at core body temperature.

Extensive clinical trials have shown the vaccine to be well tolerated in adults and children, to induce humoral, cell-mediated and secretory immune responses and to provide high levels of protective immunity against the strains of virus used in the vaccine. Cross-reactivity against strains not included in the vaccine has also been shown. The vaccine is also highly protective against variants of the vaccine HA subtype that have undergone antigenic drift, relative to the wild-type antigen.

In addition to protective efficacy rates approaching 100% in some studies of cold-adapted intranasal vaccination, the vaccine was also shown to reduce some measures of illness in vaccinated patients who became infected. For example, in one study, febrile illness and antibiotic use were reduced by 21% and 28%, respectively, in vaccinated patients, relative to placebo.

7

Vaccine standardization

Selection of strains

Virus isolates from national centres are submitted to one or more of the WHO's four collaborating centres for antigen and genetic analyses. In February of each year, the WHO recommends which viral strains should be included in the next year's vaccine for the northern hemisphere. A second review is held each September to consider whether further recommendations should be made for vaccines for the southern hemisphere. Three types of data are assessed in making the recommendation.

- **Antigenic and genetic data on recent virus isolates:** these data are compared with those of isolates obtained in the recent past
- **Epidemiological data:** to assess whether the new isolates have the potential to spread and cause disease
- **Antibody responses:** to assess the ability of currently available vaccines to evoke antibody responses to newly detected viruses

How well do the WHO recommendations work?

In the decade 1987–1997, no changes were made in the recommendation for the A/H1N1 strain, nine changes for the A/H3N2 strain and four changes for the influenza B strain. A good match was achieved in respect of 23 (77%) of 30 circulating strains but, when considered on an annual basis, the epidemic strains were antigenically different from the vaccine strains during five of 10 seasons.

Antigen content of current vaccines

Influenza vaccines are standardized using a single radial immunodiffusion test to measure the quantity of HA protein.

When this test was first developed, 7–20 µg HA was found to evoke a satisfactory immune response in primed individuals. Most vaccines in the world contain 15 µg HA of each strain and this dose has been formally standardized in the European Union.

Figure 7.2. Match between vaccine recommendations and concurrent epidemic strains			
Season	A/H1N1	A/H3N2	B
1987–1988	+	–	–
1988–1989	+	+	+
1989–1990	+	+	+
1990–1991	+	–	+
1991–1992	+	+	+
1992–1993	+	–	+
1993–1994	+	–	+
1994–1995	+	–	–
1995–1996	+	+	+
1996–1997	+	+	+

Immunogenicity studies

Since 1992, the European Union has issued requirements for harmonization of influenza vaccines, which include annual clinical trials for

7

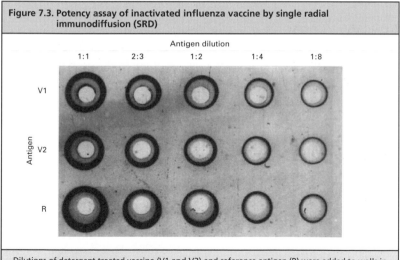

Figure 7.3. Potency assay of inactivated influenza vaccine by single radial immunodiffusion (SRD)

Dilutions of detergent treated vaccine (V1 and V2) and reference antigen (R) were added to wells in agarose gels containing sheep antiserum to influenza virus HA. SRD precipitin rings were measured and zone area was plotted against antigen dilution. Reproduced with permission from Wood JM. Standardization of inactivated influenza vaccines. In: Nicholson KG, Webster RG, Hay AJ, eds. *Textbook of Influenza*. Oxford: Blackwell Science, 1998: 333–345.

Figure 7.4. European Union criteria for the assessment of vaccines		
Criterion	**18–60 years**	**> 60 years**
Seroconversions or significant rises in anti-HA antibody titre	> 40%	> 30%
Mean geometric increase in titre	> 2.5	> 2.0
Patients achieving HAI titre > 40 or SRH titre > 25 mm^2	> 70%	> 60%
For each virus strain, at least one of the above criteria should be met.		

licensing. Regular vaccine trials are also carried out in other parts of the world.

Vaccine recommendations

Historically, recommendations on the use of influenza vaccine were based on the following.

- The concentration of influenza-associated morbidity and mortality in high-risk groups during outbreaks
- Vaccine efficacy studies in young military recruits
- Vaccine antigenicity studies

In the absence of sound scientific data, the value of immunization in high-risk groups was questioned for various reasons: outbreaks of influenza continued to be reported among the elderly, especially in nursing homes; some high-risk medical conditions (e.g. diabetes, hypertension and asthma) were being better managed than before; living standards had improved; and antimicrobial and antiviral agents were available.

Consequently, recommendations differed considerably among countries. Immunization levels were low in many countries and vaccine distribution varied markedly even among countries that had the same recommendations. Clearly, better information was needed.

Figure 7.5. Influenza immunization policies

US ACIP recommendations Target groups for special vaccination programmes	European countries with similar recommendations[a]	Policy agreement within Europe[b]
Groups at increased risk of influenzal complications		
Persons aged ≥ 65 years	17 (68%)	17 (81%)
Residents of nursing homes and long-term care facilities	15 (60%)	15 (71%)
Adults and children with chronic pulmonary disorders	21 (84%)	21 (100%)
Adults and children with chronic cardiovascular disorders	21 (84%)	21 (100%)
Adults and children who required regular medical follow-up or hospitalization during the preceding year because of:		
chronic metabolic diseases, including diabetes	18 (72%)	18 (86%)
renal dysfunction	18 (72%)	18 (86%)
haemoglobinopathies	6 (24%)	15 (71%)
immunosuppression	17 (68%)	17 (81%)
Children and teenagers on long-term aspirin therapy	6 (24%)	15 (71%)
Groups who can transmit influenza to high-risk persons		
Patients, nurses and other personnel in hospital and outpatient settings who have contact with high-risk persons; employees of nursing homes and long-term care facilities; providers of home-care to high-risk patients	15 (60%)	15 (71%)
Household members of high-risk persons	8 (32%)	13 (62%)
Other groups		
Anyone wishing to reduce chance of acquiring influenza	2 (8%)	19 (90%)
Those providing essential services	5 (20%)	16 (76%)
Students and others in institutions	1 (4%)	20 (95%)
Pregnant women with high-risk conditions	5 (20%)	16 (76%)
HIV-infected persons	6 (24%)	15 (71%)
Those travelling abroad	0 (0%)	21 (100%)

[a]Total of 25 countries for which details of recommendations were made available: Albania, Austria, Belgium, Czech Republic, Denmark, Finland, France, Germany, Greece, Hungary, Ireland, Italy, Luxembourg, Malta, Netherlands, Norway, Poland, Portugal, Romania, Slovakia, Spain, Switzerland, Sweden, Turkey, UK. [b]Total of 21 countries: immunization policies were not available from Albania, Luxembourg, Poland and Turkey. Adapted with permission from Nicholson KG, Snacken R, Palache AM. Influenza immunization policies in Europe and the USA. *Vaccine* 1995; 13: 365–369.

7

7

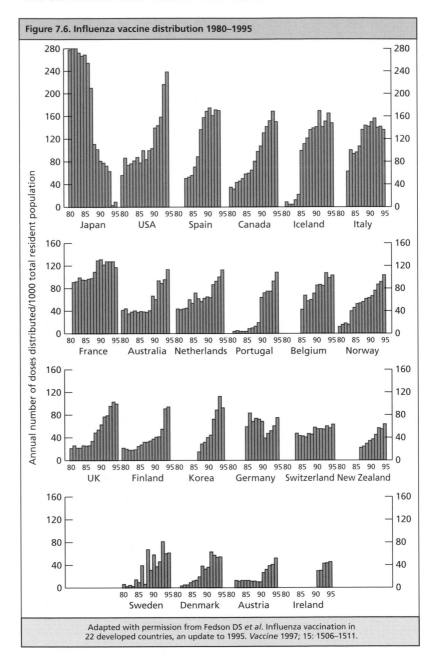

Figure 7.6. Influenza vaccine distribution 1980–1995

Adapted with permission from Fedson DS et al. Influenza vaccination in 22 developed countries, an update to 1995. Vaccine 1997; 15: 1506–1511.

Vaccine efficacy and effectiveness in elderly people

Efficacy

Few trials have studied the efficacy of influenza vaccine in the elderly. A randomized controlled trial conducted in Australia in 1969 showed that monovalent influenza vaccine was associated with a 62% reduction in laboratory-confirmed influenza illness. In Holland, a trial was held to assess vaccine efficacy in elderly people during the 1991–1992 season (when vaccine and epidemic strains were well matched). Vaccination was associated with an overall 58% reduction in clinical and laboratory-confirmed influenza.

Effectiveness

Recent studies in the USA, Canada and the UK have convincingly demonstrated the benefits of influenza vaccination in elderly people. These studies of the effectiveness of vaccination in preventing hospitalization for pneumonia and influenza, hospitalization for all respiratory conditions and deaths invariably demonstrate effectiveness, both during influenza A and B seasons and during 'non-epidemic' years.

Hospitalization for pneumonia and influenza

Vaccination is associated with 30–63% reductions in hospitalizations for pneumonia and influenza. The case–control study in a health-maintenance organization in Portland, Oregon, USA, was conducted over nine influenza seasons in the 1980s and stratified patients by risk status. The aggregate vaccine effectiveness in preventing pneumonia and influenza admissions throughout the study was 30% for high-risk elderly and 40% for low-risk elderly people. Although overall the immunization programme saved about $1 per elderly person vaccinated, these savings accrued from the vaccination of high-risk elderly patients only.

Data from Minnesota show the benefits of influenza vaccination in people with heart or lung disease (grouped as high risk), those with diabetes, renal disease, stroke, dementia or rheumatological disease (intermediate risk) and the remainder (low risk). Vaccination over six seasons was associated with an overall reduction of 39% for

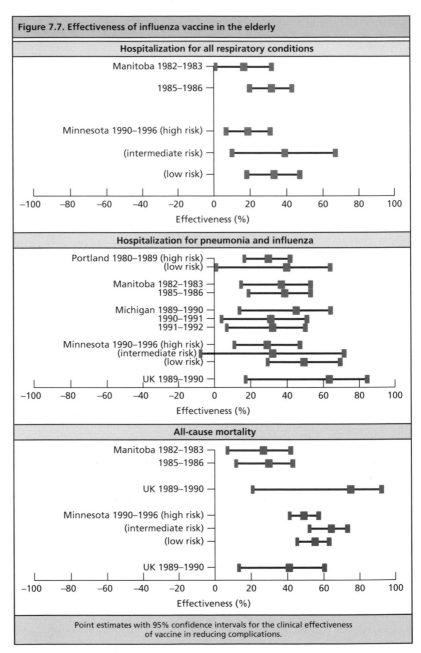

Figure 7.7. Effectiveness of influenza vaccine in the elderly

Point estimates with 95% confidence intervals for the clinical effectiveness of vaccine in reducing complications.

pneumonia hospitalizations; within the risk subgroups, the reduction was 29%, 32% and 49% for high-, intermediate- and low-risk elderly patients, respectively.

Hospitalization for all respiratory conditions

Studies in Manitoba, Canada, and Minnesota, USA, have similarly shown that influenza vaccination is associated with 17–39% reductions in hospitalizations for all respiratory conditions, with comparable levels of effectiveness in high-, intermediate- and low-risk elderly patients.

All-cause mortality and influenzal deaths

Vaccination is associated with 27–75% reductions in all-cause mortality and a 41% reduction in influenzal deaths, with similar levels of effectiveness in high-, intermediate- and low-risk elderly patients.

7

Other health gains

The following benefits have been observed during the influenza season in association with vaccination.

- An overall 27% decrease in hospitalizations for congestive cardiac failure in Minnesota between 1990 and 1996
- Reductions of 7% and 16%, respectively, for consultations for all respiratory conditions and for pneumonia and influenza in Minnesota
- A decrease of 79% in hospital admissions in people with diabetes, mostly for diabetic control, during the epidemics of 1989–1990 and 1993 in Leicester, UK

Meta-analysis

In a meta-analysis of 20 cohort observational studies of influenza vaccine in elderly patients, which span the period 1965–1989 and include epidemics caused by A/H2N2, A/H3N2 or influenza B, pooled

Figure 7.8. Reduction in complications of influenza among the elderly		
Complication	Prevention	95% CI
Respiratory illness	56%	39–68%
Pneumonia	53%	35–66%
Hospitalization	50%	28–65%
Death	68%	56–76%

estimates showed that vaccination was associated with improved outcome, assessed by reduction in respiratory illness, hospitalization and death.

Repeat vaccination

Recommendations for repeated annual vaccination arise from the changing antigenic properties of influenza virus and the decline in antibody levels from one influenza season to the next. The apparent failure of a programme of repeated annual vaccination in an English public school during 1975–1976 (when there was a poor match between vaccine and epidemic strains) raised doubts initially concerning the efficacy or effectiveness of annual revaccination.

The following studies of people vaccinated for the first time compared with those who had also been vaccinated in previous years provide no evidence for decreasing protection with repeated annual vaccination.

- In a 5-year study in Houston, the efficacy of sequential annual vaccination with a whole-virion vaccine was examined in healthy adults aged 30–60 years. Protection against infection was at least as good in multivaccinated people as in first-time vaccinees
- A case–control study in elderly people in the UK showed that, although influenza vaccination was associated with an overall reduction in mortality of 41%, the effectiveness was 75% for repeat vaccinees and only 9% for first-time vaccinees

- In a randomized, double-blind, placebo-controlled trial in elderly people in Holland during 1991–1992, the protection against clinical serologically confirmed influenza in revaccinees (89%) was twice that in first-time vaccinees (44%)

The above and several other field studies together with 12 articles on sero-response after single and multiple vaccinations have recently been subjected to meta-analyses. The analyses showed no evidence for decreasing protection with annually repeated influenza vaccination.

Figure 7.9. Efficacy of vaccination 1983–1988				
Season	Vaccine group	Epidemic virus	Efficacy (%)	
			Infection	Illness
1983–1984	First-time	H1, B	24, 70	31, 60
	Repeat		81, 75	74, 23
1984–1985	First-time	H3	65	51
	Repeat		77	66
1985–1986	First-time	B	55	37
	Repeat		56	35
1986–1987	First-time	H1	72	72
	Repeat		62	58
1987–1988	First-time	H3	49	48
	Repeat		46	34

Adapted with permission from Couch RB *et al*. Prevention of influenza virus infections by current inactivated influenza virus vaccines. In: Brown LE, Hampson AW, Webster RG, eds. *Options for the Control of Influenza III*. Amsterdam: Elsevier Science, 1996: 97–106.

Immunization of healthcare workers

Protection of high-risk populations may be improved by immunization of healthcare workers and other groups who can transmit influenza to them. The US Advisory Committee on Immunization Practices and almost two-thirds of European countries with vaccine recommendations suggest that the following groups should be vaccinated.

- Physicians, nurses and other personnel in hospital and outpatient settings
- Employees of nursing homes and long-term care facilities
- Providers of home care to persons at high risk
- Household members, including children, of persons at high risk

Attempts to increase vaccine uptake among hospital personnel have been made using a mobile cart vaccination programme. Immunization rates of 25–40% have been attained and, although influenza vaccine may reduce febrile respiratory illness and absenteeism among employees, there have been no convincing reductions in nosocomial rates of infection among patients.

Benefits of vaccination in working populations

Controlled trials carried out in Europe, North America and Australia during the 1950s and 1960s revealed that influenza vaccination is associated with reductions in work absenteeism from respiratory illness.

A recent study suggests that vaccination of healthy working adults against influenza may be highly effective. During the 1994–1995 influenza season, the benefits from vaccinating healthy working adults were examined in a double-blind, placebo-controlled trial involving 849 people; vaccination resulted in fewer complications and less disruption to the working lives of the participants.

Vaccine studies in children

Evidence shows that healthy children under 2 years old often develop inadequate antibody responses both to natural infection with influenza and after administration of one or two doses of inactivated vaccine. Current split-product vaccines have been shown to provide low levels of protection against virologically confirmed influenza in young children.

The three vaccination seasons 1985–1986, 1986–1987 and 1987–1988 provided an opportunity to assess the efficacy of influenza vaccine against infection by A/H1N1, A/H3N2 and influenza B. Efficacy was high for 10–18-year-old children (80–100%), intermediate in 6–9-year-olds (32–91%) and low for 3–5-year-olds (0–53%). All of the children were

Figure 7.10. Benefits of vaccination in workers	
Complication or disruption	Reduction (%)
Incidence of upper respiratory tract illness	25
Duration of upper respiratory tract illness	20
Sick leave due to upper respiratory tract illness	43
Consultations	44
Duration of sick leave due to all illness	36

followed for a further year without a repeat vaccination and no evidence of persistence of immunity was found in any of the three groups.

Immune-response studies

Whole-virus versus split-virus vaccines

In primed individuals (e.g. adults during interpandemic periods), whole-virus, split-virus and purified surface-antigen vaccines are considered to have equivalent antigenicity. However, some investigators have found that whole-virion vaccines may be more antigenic than split-virus vaccines in elderly primed individuals.

Concern has been voiced that split-virus and surface-antigen formulations may be less immunogenic than whole-virus vaccines in immunologically naive populations (e.g. when a new pandemic virus emerges) or in young children. Clinical trials during the 1970s, when the A/H1N1 virus re-emerged, showed that split-virus formulations of vaccine were less antigenic than whole-virus vaccines. Two doses of a split-virus vaccine were concluded to be necessary in an immunologically naive population to achieve a satisfactory response.

The effects of age

The serum HAI antibody response is generally lower in older people. The decrease in immune response can be explained partly by variations of prevaccination HAI titre, chronic ill health and possibly nutritional status but some individuals may respond poorly because of an age-related decline in immune function. The decision to immunize elderly

Figure 7.11. Efficacy of influenza vaccines among children aged 3–18 years					
Year	Vaccination[a]	Epidemic virus	Efficacy (%)		
			3–5 years	6–9 years	10–18 years
1985–1986	Yes	B	53	60[b]	80[b]
1986–1987	Yes	H1	0	32	100[b]
1987–1988	Yes	H3	27	91[b]	100[b]
1988–1989	No	H1, B	21, 35[c]	21, 35[c]	32, 0

[a]n = 131–136 children for each year; [b]$P \leq 0.05$ versus placebo; $P > 0.1$ for all others; [c]3–9-year-old children. Adapted with permission from Couch RB et al. Prevention of influenza virus infections by current inactivated influenza virus vaccines. In: Brown LE, Hampson AW, Webster RG, eds. *Options for the Control of Influenza III*. Amsterdam: Elsevier Science, 1996: 97–106.

patients should be guided by the proven effectiveness and economic benefits of vaccination rather than by the tendency for lower antibody responses with ageing.

Renal failure

Neither the efficacy nor the effectiveness of influenza vaccination have been demonstrated in people with chronic renal disease. Nonetheless, most advisory committees recommend that these patients are vaccinated. After vaccination, 50–93% (mean 67%) of patients with poor renal function achieve protective or significant rises in antibody titre to influenza A, compared with 64–94% (mean 81%) of those with normal renal function. For influenza B, 7–60% (mean 36%) of patients with poor renal function develop significant rises, compared with 50–83% (mean 61%) of those with healthy kidneys.

Transplantation

Fourfold or greater antibody responses have been documented in 30–90% of renal transplant recipients, the poorer responses occurring in patients with allograft dysfunction, uraemia and cyclosporin-induced immunosuppression. The data support recommendations to offer influenza immunization annually to these vulnerable patients.

Bone marrow transplant recipients do not respond to influenza vaccine for at least 6 months after transplantation.

The frequency of HAI antibody response by recipients of other body organs appears to be lower than that of kidney recipients. Those who are going to respond to vaccination do so after a single dose and a further injection offers little advantage.

HIV infection

HAI antibody responses to influenza vaccination decline as HIV infection progresses. Post-vaccination HAI titres of at least 1 in 64 to influenza A are found in significantly more HIV-seronegative controls (73–100%) than patients with symptomatic HIV infection (29–78%) or AIDS (24–38%). About one in eight patients with symptomatic HIV infection or AIDS responds with protective antibody levels to influenza B vaccination.

Because influenza can result in serious illness and prolonged shedding, which increases the risk of influenza to others, some national vaccine advisory committees recommend vaccination of HIV-infected patients. However, evidence suggests that patients with CD4+ cell counts of less than $300 \times 10^6/l$ are unlikely to mount influenza-specific cellular and humoral responses. A second booster dose of vaccine does not appear to improve the immune response.

Cytotoxic drug therapy

Suboptimal responses to influenza vaccine have been reported in cancer patients receiving myelosuppressive chemotherapy. Significantly fewer children and adults seroconvert when vaccinated simultaneously with chemotherapy than when vaccinated between courses of chemotherapy. In children, immunogenicity is enhanced when a period of more than 1 month has elapsed since the last chemotherapy and the leucocyte count exceeds 1000 cells/mm³. A two-dose regimen increases the antibody responses of adult lymphoma patients on chemotherapy from around 20–30% (to H1, H3 and influenza B) to around 40–50%. HAI antibody titres of at least 1 : 32 are not as effective a predictor of resistance to infection in children with cancer as in immunologically normal children.

Diabetes mellitus

No differences were found between the immune responses of patients with diabetes mellitus and healthy controls. A case–control study demonstrated that vaccination of people with diabetes can reduce hospital admissions for diabetic events and acute respiratory illness by 79%. Most advisory committees recommend vaccination for patients with diabetes.

Cystic fibrosis

In an observational study of 38 children and young adults with cystic fibrosis, HAI antibody titres were examined before and after annual influenza vaccination for 10 years. Most had post-vaccination HAI antibody titres of at least 1 : 40, with no upward or downward trend of either pre or post geometric mean antibody titres over the 10 years.

7

Adverse effects of inactivated vaccines

Many millions of doses of influenza vaccine are administered throughout the world each year and the overall rate of adverse reactions is low. Adverse events definitely associated with vaccine include local reactions, increased bronchial reactivity to histamine or methacholine in asthmatic patients and anaphylaxis. Guillain–Barré syndrome (GBS) was temporally associated with the 1976–1977 porcine influenza vaccination programme and the 1992–1993 and 1993–1994 seasons.

Local and systemic reactions

The current split-product and purified surface-antigen vaccines cause few side effects. Studies have found no systemic reactions to either product. In Spain, reactions to more than 21 000 doses of vaccine were assessed by questionnaire 1 and 2 weeks after administration. Purified surface-antigen vaccines caused the fewest local reactions and whole-virus vaccines caused most; no differences were seen in systemic reactions.

Figure 7.12. Adverse effects of inactivated influenza vaccine

Adverse effect	Frequency	Association with vaccination
Local erythema and tenderness	17–64%	Definite
Fever and systemic symptoms	2–34%	Similar to placebo
Cutaneous reactions: pemphigoid, vasculitis, dermatomyositis, Gianotti–Crosti syndrome	Case reports	Possible
Uveitis	Case report	Possible
Allergic reactions immediate or delayed anaphylaxis	Rare	Definite
fatal anaphylaxis	Case reports	Definite
Neurological problems Guillain–Barré syndrome	1 per 100 000 (1976–1977) to 1–2 per 1 000 000 vaccines (1992–1993 and 1993–1994)	Probable
meningoencephalitis	Case reports	Possible
encephalopathy	Case reports	Possible
reversible paralysis	Case reports	Possible
Exacerbation of chronic respiratory disease increased bronchial reactivity to histamine or methacholine	Up to 90% of asthmatics	Definite
clinically significant exacerbations	0–2%	Probable
Transient increase in viral load in HIV+ patients	Variable up to 90%	Probable

Adapted with permission from Wiselka MJ. Vaccination safety. In: Nicholson KG, Webster RG, Hay AJ, eds. *Textbook of Influenza*. Oxford: Blackwell Science, 1998: 346–357.

7

Guillain–Barré syndrome

An increased incidence of GBS after A/New Jersey/76 vaccination led to suspension of the national influenza immunization programme and to nationwide surveillance of the syndrome. This identified 1098 affected patients from October 1976 to January 1977, 532 of whom had received an influenza injection before onset of the syndrome. Analysis revealed an attributable risk of vaccine-related GBS of one case per 100 000 vaccinations. About 6% of affected patients died, the case-fatality increasing with age from about 1% in children to almost 13% in those aged more than 65 years.

Subsequently no increased risk of developing GBS was evident until the 1992–1993 and 1993–1994 seasons, when an overall relative risk of

1.83 was observed during the 6 weeks after vaccination. This equated to one to two cases per million vaccinees.

The potential benefits of influenza vaccination outweigh the possible risks for vaccine-associated GBS. However, because the risk of developing GBS is increased considerably in people with a history of GBS, it is prudent to avoid immunization of such individuals.

Exacerbation of asthma

Bronchoprovocation tests show increased bronchial reactivity in people with asthma for several days after vaccination against influenza and anecdotal reports suggest an association between vaccination and exacerbations. Most observational and placebo-controlled studies suggest that influenza vaccine is safe in people with asthma.

The safety of influenza vaccination in patients with asthma was recently assessed in a large double-blind, placebo-controlled, crossover study, with allowance made for the occurrence of colds, which can also exacerbate asthma. Of 255 participants with paired data, eight had a reduction in peak expiratory flow of greater than 30% after vaccination, compared with none after placebo. However, when participants with colds were excluded, no significant difference in the numbers with reductions of more than 20% was found between vaccine and placebo.

Pulmonary function abnormalities may occur as a complication of influenza vaccination but the risk is very small and is outweighed by the benefits of vaccination.

Corneal allograft rejection

Cases of corneal allograft rejection after vaccination have been reported. In one series of five vaccine-associated cases, four patients developed graft rejection within weeks of influenza vaccination.

False-positive laboratory tests

During the 1991–1992 season, vaccination was associated with the transient appearance of antibodies giving false-positive serological reactions in tests for antibodies to HIV, HTLV-I and hepatitis C virus. There is no evidence that vaccinees are at increased risk of contracting infection with any of these pathogens.

Precautions and contraindications

Allergy

Influenza vaccine is contraindicated in persons with a history of an immediate sensitivity reaction (e.g. hives, angio-oedema, bronchospasm or anaphylaxis), especially anaphylactic reactions to a previous dose, to chicken eggs or egg products or to ingredients in the vaccine formulation. Some manufacturers state that influenza vaccine is contraindicated in individuals allergic to chicken or to chicken feathers. However, patients who can eat eggs can generally receive influenza vaccine safely.

Most individuals with documented sensitivity to eggs can be vaccinated successfully with no adverse effects, provided that appropriate skin testing (with a 1 in 100 dilution of vaccine) and desensitization are carried out in a facility where immediate reactions can be treated safely. The protocol described by Murphy and Strunk (1985) provides a method of skin testing and administration of incremental doses of vaccine to those with egg allergy.

Febrile illness

Although vaccination of individuals with acute febrile illness should preferably be deferred, minor illnesses with or without fever are not contraindications, particularly in children with mild upper respiratory tract illness.

Guillain–Barré syndrome

In light of the available data, influenza immunization should be avoided in individuals with a history of GBS, especially in those who developed GBS within 6 weeks of a previous influenza vaccination.

Pregnancy

There is no evidence that influenza vaccine causes fetal damage and vaccination is considered safe in pregnant women. Vaccination is recommended in pregnant women who have a medical condition increasing their risk of complications and, in the USA, it is recommended for all pregnant women who will be in their second or third trimester during the influenza season.

Drug interactions

Increased theophylline levels have been reported after the administration of influenza vaccine, although most studies have failed to show any clinically important interaction. Similarly, there have been conflicting reports on whether influenza vaccine alters the pharmacokinetics of phenytoin or warfarin. No interaction between influenza vaccine and the antivirals amantadine and rimantadine is evident.

Other vaccines

The target groups for influenza and pneumococcal vaccination overlap. The two vaccines can be administered concurrently at separate sites without increasing the risk of adverse effects. Pneumococcal vaccine is generally given no more frequently than once every 3–5 years because of the increased incidence and severity of adverse reactions to revaccination at intervals of less than 3 years.

There have been no studies on concomitant administration of influenza vaccine, live or inactivated, with other childhood vaccines. In the USA, it has been stated that influenza vaccine may be given to children concurrently, but at separate sites, with MMR, Haemophilus b, varicella, polio and hepatitis A and B vaccines. Concern that both influenza and DTP vaccines can induce fever, which may be additive, has led to the view that infants and young children at high risk of the complications of influenza should receive acellular rather than whole-cell pertussis vaccines if administered concurrently with the influenza vaccine.

Timing of influenza immunization

Protective levels of antibody may take 10–14 days to develop. Annual programmes of immunization should be completed before the beginning of the influenza season. In temperate countries of the northern hemisphere, influenza activity typically peaks between late December and March but can often be detected beforehand. Peak activity occurs in June in New Zealand and July to August in Australia. Details of the local seasonality of influenza can be provided by the national influenza centres.

The ideal time for immunization in Europe and North America is between early October and mid-November to ensure high coverage before early outbreaks. However, early immunization risks the waning of antibodies in the frail elderly population ahead of a late epidemic. Thus, the optimal time for immunizing geriatric individuals may be November.

When available, influenza vaccination should continue to be offered to unimmunized individuals until influenza activity declines.

7

Organizing the programme

More effective immunization strategies are required to improve vaccine coverage from current suboptimal levels. Studies show that the single most important factor affecting vaccine uptake is whether the doctor or nurse recommends it. The immunization programme involves a combination of the following relevant practices.

- Labelling the notes or electronic record of persons for whom vaccination is recommended (recommendation based on chronic-disease register, e.g. asthma or diabetes, regular prescriptions for key drugs, patient's age and routine consultations throughout the year)
- Informing those patients at risk from the complications of influenza during routine contacts that they should be vaccinated during the season

- Educating supporting healthcare personnel (e.g. health visitor, receptionist, practice nurse), so that they can pass on relevant advice
- Targeting relevant educational materials at patients in at-risk groups and their carers
- Arranging and advertising immunization sessions, identifying those who should receive vaccine. Displaying pamphlets and posters in the doctor's office or surgery
- Using a computerized database to send reminder letters (or a telephone invitation) to those who are able to come to the doctor's surgery, including instructions for making alternative arrangements if the first offer is inconvenient
- Making arrangements with medical staff to immunize those who are housebound
- Making arrangements with managers of long-term care facilities well in advance for immunization of residents. Organizing consent for vaccination from next of kin, where appropriate, in advance of vaccination
- Enhancing compliance among healthcare personnel by providing convenient access to vaccine (e.g. using a mobile cart taking vaccine directly to the clinic, ward or nursing home and making vaccine available during night and weekend workshifts)

Infection control

Consideration should be given to the following to minimize the likelihood of transmission of influenza in residential care facilities or hospitals.

Patients

- Patients with uncomplicated influenza and without features of concern requiring urgent hospitalization should not be admitted to hospital
- In hospital, newly admitted patients with influenza-like illness of less than 5 days' duration and patients who develop nosocomial influenza while hospitalized require 'respiratory

isolation'. They should be nursed in isolation for up to 5 days after onset of illness. Patients with influenzal complications are not necessarily admitted during the early stages of influenza when viral shedding is at its peak and may not need isolation
- In residential care facilities, residents with influenza-like illness should be isolated or cohorted, preferably for up to 5 days after onset. The use of amantadine or rimantadine in the index case may risk transmission of drug-resistant virus if index and non-infected residents are allowed to mix. Ongoing studies should reveal whether the NA inhibitors should be considered as an alternative

Staff

- Strong consideration should be given to annual immunization of all medical, nursing and other personnel in contact with high-risk patients and providers of home care, as recommended in many countries
- During an epidemic, prophylactic use of antivirals should be considered for unimmunized hospital personnel and other carers
- Staff with influenza-like illness should not attend work while acutely ill
- Whenever possible, only staff who have been vaccinated, who have had confirmed influenza or who are taking antiviral prophylaxis should care for infected patients
- During outbreaks in residential care facilities, movement of staff (and patients) from one ward to another should be avoided
- Staff should be reminded of the need to be vigilant in identifying patients and residents who develop influenza-like illness and notify them to the infection control personnel

Visitors

- Visitors with respiratory illness should be discouraged and consideration should be given to restricting entry of visitors with respiratory illness to patients with high-risk conditions, especially the immunocompromised
- Visitors should be informed of the isolation procedures

7

If vaccination has been given late and the risk of infection is relatively high, a concomitant course of antivirals is recommended to reduce the likelihood of infection during the 2-week period after vaccination, when protective antibody levels are reached.

7

CHAPTER 8

Treatment and prophylaxis

- Symptomatic relief is focused on reduction of fever, pain relief and rehydration; cough suppression is not recommended
- Influenza is occasionally complicated by secondary bacterial pneumonia; treatment therefore may involve empirical therapy with antibiotics
- Treatment with antivirals is recommended in outbreaks among high-risk groups, such as nursing-home residents
- Amantadine and rimantadine have some use in the treatment and prophylaxis of influenza, although both drugs cause side effects, have a propensity to induce resistant strains and are inactive against influenza B
- NA inhibitors, a new class of anti-influenza drugs (the first of which is zanamivir), are becoming available. These agents are effective against influenza A and B, are not associated with clinical resistance at levels seen with amantadine and rimantadine and are well tolerated

8

Introduction

Nearly all acute respiratory illness is viral in origin. Until recently, no specific treatment for most of these infections was available and patients have been conditioned to stay at home and treat their own symptoms. Antivirals against influenza have been available since 1966 but, outside the USA and the former Soviet Union, the use of amantadine (Symmetrel®) and rimantadine (Flumadine®) has been limited, largely because of side effects, lack of perceived benefits and propensity for induction of drug-resistant viral strains. NA inhibitors, a new class of antivirals for influenza, have shown considerable promise in clinical trials and are now available in several countries. The first NA inhibitor, zanamivir (Relenza®), is expected to become widely available during 1999, with at least one other agent in advanced stages of clinical development.

Symptomatic relief

Salicylates, once commonly used to treat influenza, are contraindicated because of the association with Reye's syndrome particularly in children. Acetaminophen (paracetamol) is recommended because of its analgesic and antipyretic properties; it may also decrease oxygen demands, discomfort and fluid loss associated with fever.

Cough suppressants may enable rest but they interfere with clearance of secretions during the early stage, when ciliary function is severely impaired, and are probably best avoided. The anticholinergic nasal spray ipratropium bromide inhibits nasal secretions and may have a role in influenza. Nasal congestion can be relieved by intranasal oxymetazoline or phenylephrine.

Antimicrobials

8

Influenza can be difficult to distinguish from other viral respiratory infections and doctors must also consider whether patients with influenzal symptoms have secondary bacterial or community-acquired pneumonia requiring treatment with antibiotics. With increasing antimicrobial resistance, the use of empirical antibiotics in community-acquired upper respiratory tract infections is a concern because half of the clinical antimicrobial use is for infections at this site and most of these infections are viral.

Most influenzal infections are uncomplicated and do not require antibiotics. Tracheitis and tracheobronchitis are the most common lower respiratory tract complications of influenza and trials of antibiotic administration in acute bronchitis have not shown a clinically important benefit of treatment.

Chronic obstructive airways disease is frequently exacerbated by influenza but the benefit of antibiotic treatment is modest and the British Thoracic Society recommends antibiotic therapy only when any two of the following three features are present: worsening dyspnoea, increased sputum volume and increased sputum purulence.

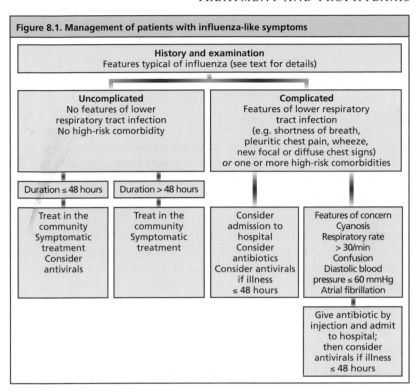

Figure 8.1. Management of patients with influenza-like symptoms

History and examination
Features typical of influenza (see text for details)

Uncomplicated	Complicated
No features of lower respiratory tract infection No high-risk comorbidity	Features of lower respiratory tract infection (e.g. shortness of breath, pleuritic chest pain, wheeze, new focal or diffuse chest signs) or one or more high-risk comorbidities

Duration ≤ 48 hours	Duration > 48 hours		
Treat in the community Symptomatic treatment Consider antivirals	Treat in the community Symptomatic treatment	Consider admission to hospital Consider antibiotics Consider antivirals if illness ≤ 48 hours	Features of concern Cyanosis Respiratory rate > 30/min Confusion Diastolic blood pressure ≤ 60 mmHg Atrial fibrillation

Give antibiotic by injection and admit to hospital; then consider antivirals if illness ≤ 48 hours

Acute otitis media is a common finding in young children with influenza; antibiotics are probably unnecessary.

Some patients with influenza-like illness have evidence of lower respiratory tract involvement and should be considered for antibiotics in the community setting; others require admission to hospital. Unnecessary hospital admission is to be discouraged, however, because it can result in nosocomial infection in high-risk patients. Antibiotic treatment should not be delayed if pneumonia is suspected.

Secondary bacterial pneumonia occurring as a complication of influenza is usually caused by *Staphylococcus aureus* but *Streptococcus pneumoniae*, *Haemophilus influenzae*, Gram-negative and mixed infections are not uncommon. Staphylococcal pneumonia is associated with rapid deterioration.

The different causes of community-acquired pneumonia, including those complicating influenza, cannot be distinguished, so antibiotics should be selected to cover the likely pathogens. The antibiotic regimen should always include a drug with activity against *S. pneumoniae*, the most common cause of community-acquired pneumonia, but, during outbreaks of influenza, cover should also be directed at *S. aureus*.

Amantadine and rimantadine

The parent compound, 1-amino-adamantane hydrochloride, was discovered, in the 1960s, to inhibit replication of strains of influenza A. Numerous derivatives have been synthesized but none has a better safety and antiviral profile than rimantadine.

Antiviral activity

Both amantadine and rimantadine inhibit human A/H1N1, A/H2N2 and A/H3N2 subtypes. Non-human subtypes of influenza A are also sensitive and future variants, including pandemic strains, will almost certainly be susceptible. Neither agent inhibits influenza B.

Resistance

Resistance occurs readily with amantadine and rimantadine. All naturally occurring type A viruses are probably mixtures of sensitive and resistant strains, the latter becoming selected for during amantadine therapy. Drug-resistant strains of virus have cross-resistance between amantadine and rimantadine and no data suggest that either one is more likely to select for resistance than the other.

Resistant strains have been recovered from about one third of adults and children receiving treatment and have been identified in nursing homes where drug has been given for both treatment and prophylaxis. Resistant virus has been detected within 24–48 hours in adults, including the elderly. Although no evidence indicates that resistant viruses cause more morbidity than sensitive isolates, rimantadine recipients who shed resistant virus tend to recover more slowly than those shedding sensitive virus.

Pharmacokinetics

In young and elderly adults, peak plasma concentrations are approximately 2.5 times greater after amantadine than after rimantadine treatment. Although the plasma drug concentrations in patients with and without adverse responses to treatment overlap considerably, concentrations of both drugs are related to adverse effects and the differences in plasma concentrations after equivalent doses may explain the relative increase in adverse reactions after amantadine.

Amantadine is excreted renally, whereas rimantadine is extensively metabolized by the liver (approximately 65%) and kidney (20%) and is also excreted as unchanged drug by the kidney. The plasma half-life of amantadine is prolonged in patients with impaired renal function. The half-life of amantadine in elderly men after multiple doses is almost double that in young men. Less than 5% of the dose is removed by haemodialysis and average half-lives of 8.3 and 13 days have been recorded in patients on long-term haemodialysis. Care must be taken to ensure that the drug does not accumulate to toxic levels.

The half-life of rimantadine is prolonged in end-stage renal failure and increases with age but to a lesser extent than that of amantadine. The single-dose pharmacokinetics of rimantadine are not altered by chronic stable liver disease.

8

Adverse effects

Reports of side effects from amantadine and rimantadine have been generated largely from studies of healthy volunteers. Comparative studies indicate that rimantadine is better tolerated than amantadine at equivalent doses. In placebo-controlled studies, mild CNS side effects and gastrointestinal symptoms are increased slightly over placebo and the nature of adverse reactions to both agents are similar.

Minor neurological symptoms include insomnia, light-headedness, difficulty in concentration, nervousness, dizziness and headache. Convulsions, reported at therapeutic doses of both amantadine and rimantadine, appear to be related to drug levels.

Other adverse effects include anorexia, nausea, vomiting, dry mouth, constipation, abdominal pain and urinary retention. Side effects of amantadine and rimantadine arise mostly during the first 3–4 days of treatment and are reversible when the drug is discontinued or the dosage is reduced.

Side effects associated with amantadine have been observed most often among the elderly and people with renal insufficiency or seizure disorders. A reduced dose of amantadine ($\leq$ 100 mg daily) in elderly people and those with renal dysfunction (creatinine clearance $\leq$ 50 ml/min) is recommended. Guidelines for amantadine dosage based on creatinine clearance are found in the drug data sheet.

In one placebo-controlled study in nursing homes, rimantadine 200 mg daily was associated with increased nausea (33% versus 6%) and anxiety (50% versus 18%) and serum levels were nearly three times higher than in younger individuals. By contrast, a larger placebo-controlled study in nursing homes in Michigan, USA, showed no statistically significant differences in the frequencies of gastrointestinal or CNS symptoms between the groups receiving rimantadine 100 mg or 200 mg daily or placebo; however, patients with significant renal or hepatic disease were excluded from that study. It is therefore recommended that elderly nursing-home residents should be given rimantadine at a dose of 100 mg daily. A reduction in dosage to 100 mg daily is also recommended for adults with severe hepatic dysfunction or a creatinine clearance rate of 10 ml/min or less.

Clinical role

Both amantadine and rimantadine have been used in the prevention and treatment of influenza A for short periods during known outbreaks. They have been evaluated in studies of seasonal prophylaxis, post-exposure prophylaxis in the family setting, outbreak control in residential care and therapy of influenzal illness.

Seasonal prophylaxis

Amantadine and rimantadine are equally effective in adults and children in preventing influenza A virus infection, both in the community and in institutional settings. Seasonal prophylaxis is somewhat more effective in preventing influenza-like illness (overall efficacy ~80%)

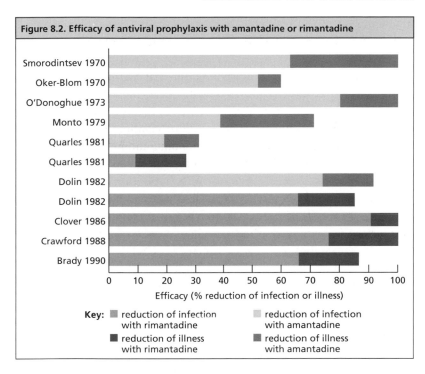

Figure 8.2. Efficacy of antiviral prophylaxis with amantadine or rimantadine

Key: ■ reduction of infection with rimantadine   ▨ reduction of infection with amantadine
■ reduction of illness with rimantadine   ■ reduction of illness with amantadine

8

than infection (~60%). This distinction may be desirable because sub-clinical infection could confer immunity against a subsequent exposure.

Post-exposure prophylaxis in households

When taken by household contacts after onset of influenza in the family, amantadine and rimantadine reduced virologically confirmed influenzal illness by 74% and 70%, respectively. However, when these drugs were used to treat index cases and contacts simultaneously, neither was effective. Failure of prophylaxis was associated with recovery of drug-resistant strains of virus from index cases and contacts treated with rimantadine.

Outbreak control in residential care

The US Advisory Committee on Immunization Practices strongly recommends that, whenever an outbreak of type A influenza is detected in a nursing home, all residents who do not have specific contraindications, whatever their immunization status, be given either amantadine or rimantadine. This recommendation is based on the known effectiveness of the two antivirals, rather than on controlled trials in outbreak situations. However, co-administration of drug for treatment and prophylaxis in residential care can lead to resistance and possibly to failure of prophylaxis. Indeed, the emergence and possible transmission of amantadine-resistant viruses in nursing homes after implementation of index case treatment and amantadine prophylaxis has been documented on several occasions.

In one report of an outbreak of influenza A infection, around 13% of residents were affected, even though 91% had received the drug. In another home, in which amantadine treatment and prophylaxis (37% coverage) was initiated but the index case was isolated, no further cases developed. Therefore the success of amantadine treatment and prophylaxis protocols may be due in part to cohorting or isolation of cases.

The optimal use of amantadine and rimantadine in controlling outbreaks requires the early identification of possible cases of influenza. The clinical picture of influenza is variable in the elderly but antiviral prophylaxis is recommended when a cluster of patients – defined as three or more on a unit during a 48–72 hour period – present with an influenza-like illness – defined as fever ($\geq 38°C$ oral) and at least one of cough, sore throat and runny or stuffy nose – during the influenza season. Ideally, at least one resident should have influenza A confirmed virologically.

Chemoprophylaxis of all residents of the affected facility should begin as soon as possible to reduce the spread of infection. Contingency planning is essential and the following activities are suggested.

- Implementing surveillance system during the influenza season to detect cases of influenza-like illness
- Collecting specimens for rapid diagnostic testing. Supplies of nasopharyngeal swabs and virus transport media should be available in the facility. Arrangements should be in place for specimen transport, rapid laboratory testing and speedy communication of the results

- Obtaining pre-approved medication orders (prescriptions) or ensuring the ability to obtain sufficient medication at short notice. Ideally, before each influenza season, the care facility should maintain sufficient drug to initiate mass prophylaxis
- Obtaining information before the influenza season on each patient's renal function to predetermine the dosage of amantadine after consulting the manufacturer's package insert. Dosage reduction for rimantadine is recommended for persons with severe renal impairment
- Offering prophylaxis to unvaccinated staff providing patient care
- Continuing surveillance in the home to identify treatment failures and emergence of resistant virus, the occurrence of adverse drug reactions and the absence of new culture-confirmed influenza in the residents
- Continuing antiviral chemoprophylaxis for at least 2 weeks or until approximately 1 week after the end of the outbreak

Treatment

8

Both amantadine and rimantadine are effective therapeutic agents in naturally occurring influenza A infection in adults and children without high-risk conditions. Administration of either agent within 48 hours of symptom onset ameliorates illness, compared with placebo. The effects on fever and on symptoms equate to a reduction in the duration of illness of about 24 hours. The duration or titre of virus excreted in upper-airway secretions decreases more rapidly in amantadine- or rimantadine-treated adults.

Whether amantadine or rimantadine can prevent the progression of uncomplicated influenza to pneumonia or whether they ameliorate the illness is not known. A significant proportion of immunocompromised patients treated with amantadine or rimantadine alone develop resistant strains, which may be shed for prolonged periods.

Neuraminidase inhibitors

Zanamivir, the first of a new class of specific, rationally designed anti-influenza agents – the NA inhibitors – has recently become available in some countries (Sweden and Australia), with extensive availability expected during 1999 and 2000. The NA inhibitors act by inhibiting the action of viral NA, which is responsible for liberating new virus particles from infected airway cells.

Zanamivir, formerly known as GG 167, has been shown to be a potent inhibitor of all strains of influenza A and B. Zanamivir does not cross cell membranes readily and is therefore not absorbed from the gastrointestinal tract. For this reason, the agent is delivered directly to the site of infection and viral replication in the airway using an inhaler.

Another NA inhibitor (GS 4104) is in late clinical development; this drug appears comparable to zanamivir in terms of *in vitro* potency, although it is given orally.

Resistance

Influenza viruses with reduced sensitivity to the NA inhibitors have been isolated after *in vitro* passaging studies. Resistance to NA inhibitors can develop in two ways: change in the NA and change in the HA. A low incidence (approximately 1%) of drug-resistant virus has been reported from two treatment studies with GS 4104, whereas no clinical isolates with reduced sensitivity to zanamivir have been seen to date in the phase II or phase III treatment studies. During prolonged treatment with zanamivir (2 weeks), a virus with mutations affecting first the HA and then the NA was recovered from a young immunocompromised child with influenza B, who was treated on a compassionate use basis.

Changes in the neuraminidase

Mutations have been detected in the NA gene, although the active site is highly conserved in the NA and this may mean a reduced propensity for this class of drug to induce resistant strains. The NA active site is largely internalized within the molecule and is therefore not exposed to the host's neutralizing antibodies. This lack of selective pressure from the host has allowed the active site to become highly conserved and therefore a very good rational target for antiviral therapy. Mutations in the NA active site induced *in vitro* tend to result in destabilization of the enzyme and thus in reduced pathogenicity of the virus.

Changes in the haemagglutinin

Most resistant viruses generated *in vitro* have a mutation in the HA that probably reduces the binding of the HA with its cell receptor. As a result, the virus is able to dissociate from infected cells with a reduced need for NA activity, although it suffers the disadvantage of weaker binding during infection. Several variants have been shown to have cross-resistance to more than one NA inhibitor.

Changes involving both the NA and the HA also occur, leading to additive effects on resistance *in vitro*. The clinical significance of such mutations remains to be determined.

Pharmacokinetics

Zanamivir is not readily absorbed after oral administration and is therefore administered by oral inhalation topically to the upper and lower airways as a dry powder via a Diskhaler™ device. Systemic exposure in healthy people is estimated at 10% after intranasal administration as drops, 20% after administration by nebulizer and 15% after inhalation of powder. These low systemic absorption figures mean that no dosage adjustment is required in renally impaired, hepatically impaired or elderly patients. The half-life after intranasal administration and inhalation is approximately 3.5 hours. Antiviral activity is readily detectable for 9 hours after intranasal administration. Almost all intravenously administered zanamivir is eliminated renally as unchanged drug.

Oral absorption of GS 4104 is approximately 70% in rats and marmosets and somewhat higher in humans. The ester prodrug (GS 4104) is absorbed and converted rapidly to the active metabolite (GS 4071), which reaches peak levels within 2–3 hours in humans. Bioavailability of the drug is affected minimally by food. The pharmacokinetic profile in healthy elderly people, including the elimination half-life, is similar

8

to that in young people, although overall exposure of the active metabolite at steady state is approximately 25% higher than in the young. The drug is eliminated primarily by renal excretion of the active metabolite, with less than 5% being recovered as unchanged prodrug. Exposure to the active compound increases with decreasing creatinine clearance and is up to fourfold higher in patients with creatinine clearance rates of 30–60 ml/min and 10-fold higher when the rate is less than 30 ml/min. The drug is not metabolized significantly by the liver and has a low degree of binding to plasma proteins.

Efficacy

Placebo-controlled studies of the prophylactic and therapeutic efficacy of zanamivir and GS 4104 have been carried out in healthy volunteers inoculated with influenza virus and in large phase III trials in people with naturally acquired influenza or who were exposed to influenza in the community.

Healthy volunteer challenge studies

When intranasal zanamivir (3.6–16 mg) was given two to six times daily to susceptible healthy volunteers, beginning 4 hours before inoculation with influenza A/Texas/91 H1N1 and continued for 5 days, the agent was 82% effective in preventing laboratory evidence of infection and 95% effective in preventing febrile illness. Comparable efficacy was observed when the drug was given once daily or intravenously.

Oral GS 4104 100 mg once or twice daily, given to susceptible healthy volunteers beginning 26 hours before virus inoculation with A/Texas/91 H1N1 and continued for 5 days, was 61% effective in preventing laboratory evidence of infection.

Early treatment with zanamivir 16 mg two or six times daily, starting 26 or 32 hours after infection with A/Texas/91 H1N1 and continued for 4 days, reduced the duration of virus shedding by a median of 3 days, the viral titre area under the curve by 87% and the peak titre by 99%. In addition, early treatment reduced the occurrence of febrile illness ($\geq 37.8°C$) by 84% and was associated with significant reductions in symptom scores.

Early treatment with GS 4104 20, 100 or 200 mg twice daily or 200 mg once daily, starting 28 hours after infection with A/Texas/91 H1N1 and continued for 5 days, reduced the duration of viral shedding by a median of 2 days and the viral titre area under the curve by 71% and was associated with significant reduction in time to alleviation of illness.

Natural influenza: prophylaxis

NA inhibitors have been shown to be effective as a prophylaxis against naturally acquired influenza.

Zanamivir was tested in a phase III trial of 1107 healthy adults who were randomized to receive either zanamivir 10 mg once daily or placebo for 4 weeks, during a period when the circulating influenza strain was known to differ from the strain included in that year's vaccine. The trial showed that zanamivir was 67% effective in preventing laboratory-confirmed symptomatic influenza and 84% effective in preventing laboratory-confirmed influenza with fever, compared with placebo.

GS 4104 was also shown during the same winter season to be effective at preventing community-acquired influenza infection. The trial involved 1559 healthy adults who were randomized into three groups, receiving either GS 4104 75 mg once or twice daily or placebo for 6 weeks. The primary endpoint was laboratory-confirmed symptomatic influenza infection, with fever of 37.2°C or more. The overall protective efficacy was 74%, with no additional benefit from the twice-daily over the once-daily protocol, relative to the placebo arm.

Natural influenza: treatment

The clinical development of NA inhibitors has involved extensive clinical trials in patients with influenza and required careful design so that the effects of these new agents on community-acquired influenza could be measured accurately.

Zanamivir was shown to be effective in the treatment of influenza in a number of multicentre, randomized clinical trials in the northern and southern hemispheres, during winter seasons when influenza was known to be circulating in the community. Similar trials have also shown the potential of GS 4104 in treating natural influenza. Throughout trials for both NA inhibitors, the primary endpoint was time to alleviation of clinically significant symptoms of influenza. Entry criteria for the zanamivir trials were fever of 37.8°C or more plus two symptoms from the following: headache, cough, myalgia and sore throat. In some studies, feverishness could substitute for fever. For GS 4104, the criteria for entry were fever of 38°C or more plus one local symptom, such as cough, sore throat or nasal symptoms, plus one systemic symptom, such as feverishness, malaise, headache and myalgia or prostration. Patients were required to present no more than 36 hours after the onset of symptoms in the GS 4104 studies and one of the zanamivir studies and within 48 hours of onset in the other zanamivir studies.

Zanamivir

Several phase II trials were conducted to compare different delivery routes and dosing frequencies of zanamivir. These trials included both orally inhaled and intranasal formulations of the agent. The intranasal formulation appeared to provide no additional benefit over the inhaled formulation alone. In addition, there was no evidence that zanamivir administered four times daily was more efficacious than zanamivir administered twice daily. In all subsequent studies, therefore, zanamivir has been given as 10 mg twice daily by oral inhalation.

The first phase III trial for zanamivir was conducted in the southern hemisphere by the MIST study group and involved 455 patients, who were randomized to receive zanamivir 10 mg twice daily for 5 days or placebo. For this trial, fever or feverishness (i.e. no measurable pyrexia but subjective feeling of chills) was used as entry criteria, although, in subsequent phase III trials of zanamivir, fever of 37.8°C or more was required for inclusion. The MIST trial showed that, compared with placebo, zanamivir relieved influenza symptoms a median of 1.5 days earlier in the intention-to-treat and influenza-positive populations and 2.0 days earlier in patients who were febrile at entry. In the subgroup of high-risk patients treated with zanamivir, symptoms were alleviated a median of 2.5 days earlier, fewer patients had complications (14% versus 46%) and fewer used complication-associated antibiotics (14% versus 38%).

The MIST study results were confirmed in further trials, including one in Europe, which also showed a reduced duration and severity of influenza symptoms. In patients with confirmed influenza, alleviation of symptoms occurred after a median of 5 days for zanamivir,

8

Figure 8.3. Efficacy data for zanamivir-treated patients

Trial	Patients (n)	Duration of illness before treatment (hours)	Reduction in duration of illness (median days)	Difference versus placebo (%)
Phase II trials				
USA/Europe (Hayden et al., N Engl J Med 1997)[a]				
ITT	417	≤ 48	0.7[b]	12
IP	262	≤ 48	1	20
IP, early presentation	130	≤ 30	3	43
USA/Europe (Monto et al., J Infect Dis 1999 in press)[c]				
ITT	1256	≤ 48	1	14
ITT, early presentation	731	≤ 30	1–1.5	15–23
IP	722	≤ 48	1.5	21
High-risk patients	158	≤ 48	1.5–2.75	19–35
Phase III trials				
Southern hemisphere (MIST study group, Lancet 1998)				
ITT	422	≤ 36	1.5	23
IP	321	≤ 36	1.5	25
IP, febrile patients (≥38.7°C)	203	≤ 36	2.0	31
High-risk patients	76	≤ 36	2.5	31
Europe (Fleming et al., IDSA, Denver, USA, 1998)				
ITT	356	≤ 48	2.5	33
IP	277	≤ 48	2.5	33
High-risk patients	32	≤ 48	2.5	22

ITT, intention-to-treat population; IP, influenza-positive population.
[a] This trial included an arm in which patients received an intranasal spray formulation of zanamivir (not being developed commercially) in addition to the orally inhaled formulation. The efficacy data presented relate only to the orally inhaled formulation (ITT n = 132, IP n = 85, IP subgroup n = 43) versus placebo, although combined use of the two formulations yielded similar results.
[b] Mean days.
[c] All patients in this trial received both orally inhaled and intranasal zanamivir or matching placebo either twice or four times daily. Efficacy data are presented for all patients receiving zanamivir versus placebo.

8

compared with 7.5 days for placebo, a reduction of 2.5 days. This reduction was seen in both the intention-to-treat and influenza-positive populations. Severity of the main symptoms of influenza infection was also reduced.

A third study (as yet unpublished) conducted in North America, confirmed the therapeutic efficacy of zanamivir: time to alleviation of major symptoms was reduced from 6 to 5 days in patients with virologically confirmed influenza infection.

Combined analysis of these three studies shows reductions in complications and associated antibiotic prescriptions.

Figure 8.4. Efficacy data for GS 4104-treated patients				
Trial	Patients (*n*)	Duration of illness before treatment (hours)	Reduction in duration of illness (median days)	Difference versus placebo (%)
Treanor *et al.*, ICAAC, 1998				
ITT	629	≤ 36	–	–
IP	374	≤ 36	1.4[a,b]	30
Aoki *et al.*, ICAAC, 1998				
ITT	719	≤ 36	–	–
IP	475	≤ 36	1.2[a]	25
			1.4[b]	30

ITT, intention-to-treat population; IP, influenza-positive population.
High-risk patients were not recruited in these studies.
[a]Patients received GS 4104 75 mg twice daily.   [b]Patients received GS 4104 150 mg twice daily.

GS 4104

GS 4104 has also been shown to be effective as a treatment for influenza infection, with reductions in duration of symptoms and complications. GS 4104 was assessed in phase II/III trials in North America and in 11 countries worldwide, including Canada, China and several European countries. Both studies showed that GS 4104 75 mg or 150 mg twice daily for 5 days was effective at reducing the severity of the major symptoms of influenza. Duration of illness was reduced by 1.4 days compared with placebo in the North American study (a median of 2.9 days of illness for the 75 mg and 150 mg dosages, compared with 4.3 days for placebo). In the international study, duration of illness was reduced by 1.2 days with the 75 mg dosage and by 1.4 days with the 150 mg dosage, compared with placebo. Further analysis of the North American data indicated that secondary influenza complications, such as bronchitis and sinusitis, were reduced by about 50% in these previously healthy adult patients. Little difference between the 75 mg and 150 mg dosages was seen in terms of efficacy.

In addition, combined analysis of these two studies and a third study (as yet unpublished) conducted in the southern hemisphere confirms the above findings and shows further that the benefit from GS 4104 was associated with a reduction in the instances of complications and the need for antibiotic therapy.

Future studies

More detailed studies are in progress to assess the efficacy of zanamivir and GS 4104 in the treatment of influenza infection in high-risk patients, including the elderly (especially those in care homes), children and patients with chronic obstructive airways disease.

Tolerability

Zanamivir was exceptionally well tolerated in all trials, with an adverse event profile that was indistinguishable from that of placebo.

Tolerability of GS 4104 was generally good, with adverse events occurring at a rate comparable to that of placebo for events other than nausea and vomiting; these were seen at a frequency exceeding that of placebo in the studies described above but appear to be ameliorated by taking the drug with food (unpublished data).

After so many years with no major advances in the control of influenza, the impending availability of a new class of antivirals offers an exciting new approach for the treatment and prophylaxis of influenza. The rationally designed NA inhibitors are likely to revolutionize the treatment of influenza because they shorten the duration of illness, allow patients to return to normal activity more quickly and appear to prevent complications.

8

CHAPTER 9

Planning for the next pandemic

- Pandemics are highly unpredictable, in terms of when and where one will occur next. The clinical characteristics, demographics, attack rates, morbidity, duration and extent vary enormously
- Planning for pandemics is carried out at the global (WHO), national (government and health service) and local levels
- Planning should follow a phased structure, beginning in the interpandemic period (phase 0), through identification of a novel virus with pandemic potential (preparedness levels 1–3) to confirmation of a global pandemic (phase 1)

Introduction

Pandemics are highly unpredictable. They occur at irregular intervals and are just as likely to be first recognized in the spring or summer as in the autumn or winter months. Attack rates, severity of illness and mortality vary enormously between pandemics and between waves of the same pandemic. Viruses with pandemic potential may fail to spread despite causing severe complications and death locally.

Most pandemics originated in the Far East, where dense populations of humans, pigs and ducks living in close proximity provide the perfect environment for genetic reassortment. However, although history suggests China as the source of the next pandemic, it could arise anywhere, with little time to prepare. The only certainty is that the new millennium will bring at least one pandemic of influenza.

When pandemics occur, they spread rapidly and, although some places remain unscathed for months, increasing international movement of people, rapid means of transportation and the opening up of tourism to China and elsewhere in Southeast Asia can be expected to shorten the time taken for the new virus to spread worldwide. Early

9

spread of a new virus could be missed in countries where influenza surveillance is not well developed.

The disruption from pandemics is enormous and the need for greater preparedness has been the subject of discussion at recent international meetings. The WHO, the USA, Canada, the UK, some other European countries and Japan are either updating or developing pandemic plans or are re-evaluating them in response to the outbreak of 'bird flu' in Hong Kong. The following have emerged as key elements of planning.

At the international level (WHO)

1. Recognizing promptly the emergence of a potential pandemic strain of virus
2. Assessing risk from a new virus by monitoring its course and seeking additional information on transmissibility, attack rates and severity
3. Isolating the virus into substrates acceptable for developing vaccines
4. Assessing sensitivity of the new strain to antiviral drugs
5. Determining prevalence of antibodies to the HA of the new virus
6. Genetic and antigenic analyses
7. Preparing and disseminating reagents for virus identification and vaccine manufacture
8. Developing and evaluating candidate vaccines
9. Distributing candidate vaccine strains to vaccine manufacturers
10. Co-ordinating clinical trials to identify most efficient use of vaccine
11. Providing information to national authorities and the media about the virus, its spread, high-risk groups, potential for control and case-management
12. Assessing the pandemic and identifying means to improve preparedness for the future

9

Phasing the response to an emerging pandemic

Common to the development of most pandemic plans is an outline of actions broadly related to the activity of the novel virus. At an international level, this can be divided into six phases: preparedness levels 1, 2 and 3 of the interpandemic period (Phase 0), corresponding to first recovery of a novel virus from one person, recovery from two or more people and a localized outbreak with person-to-person spread; onset of a pandemic (Phase 1); regional and multi-regional epidemics (Phase 2); end of first pandemic wave (Phase 3); second or later waves (Phase 4); and end of the pandemic (Phase 5).

Figure 9.1. Phased approach to pandemic planning	
Source	Action
Phase 0 Preparedness level 1 *A novel virus subtype has been recovered from a single human case, without evidence of spread or outbreak activity*	The WHO co-ordinates work to identify the source of exposure and the antibody responses to those potentially exposed to the virus, examines the virus genome, evaluates sensitivity to antiviral agents and heightens surveillance
Phase 0 Preparedness level 2 *Two or more human infections have been established but the ability to spread rapidly and cause outbreaks remains questionable*	The WHO announces Preparedness level 2, enhances virological surveillance and diagnosis, develops a case definition to study transmission and impact and promotes sero-surveys and the development and evaluation of vaccine candidates and reagents
Phase 0 Preparedness level 3 *Person-to-person spread has occurred in the general population, with at least one outbreak lasting ≥ 2 weeks in one country* or *identification of a new virus subtype in several countries*	Before announcement, the WHO excludes other possible explanations for the virological findings and establishes the potential of the virus to cause lower respiratory tract disease. The WHO disseminates a case definition for surveillance, distributes candidate vaccine viruses, develops clinical trials of vaccines against the new strain and makes recommendations for their use, disseminates information on the status of investigations of the new virus, its spread and the response to it and provides general guidance to national health authorities

9

Continued	
Source	**Action**
Phase 1 *Confirmation of onset of pandemic, i.e. new virus subtype has caused several outbreaks in one country and has spread to other countries, with disease patterns indicating that serious morbidity and mortality are likely in at least one segment of the population. Depending on the amount of early warning, this Phase may or may not have been preceded by the above levels of preparedness*	The WHO announces a new influenza pandemic, recommends the composition and use of vaccines (dose and schedule), issues guidance on the best use of available antiviral agents and further enhances monitoring and reporting of global spread
Phase 2 *Outbreaks are occurring in several countries and spreading region by region across the world*	The WHO announces the onset of Phase 2, monitors and reports the global spread and impact of the virus, organizes distribution of vaccines in the most equitable manner possible and updates information on the best use of available antiviral agents
Phase 3 *End of first pandemic wave in the initially affected countries or regions but outbreaks are still occurring elsewhere*	The WHO announces the onset of Phase 3, continues to monitor and report the global spread and impact of the virus, continues to organize distribution of vaccines and updates guidance on the best use of available antiviral agents
Phase 4 *Occurrence of second or later waves of the pandemic*	The WHO announces Phase 4, continues to monitor and report the global spread of the virus and estimates the remaining needs for vaccines and availability of antiviral agents
Phase 5 *End of the pandemic, i.e. return to Phase 0, when indices of influenza activity have returned to essentially normal interpandemic levels and immunity to the virus is widespread in the general population. Major epidemics are not expected until antigenic variants (i.e. drift) begin to emerge from the pandemic strain*	The WHO declares the end of the pandemic and the onset of the interpandemic phase (Phase 0). The WHO then assesses the overall impact of the pandemic, evaluates lessons learned that will assist in responding to future pandemics and updates the Pandemic Plan

Adapted from WHO Influenza Pandemic Preparedness Plan: Responding to an influenza pandemic or its threat – the role of WHO and guidelines for national or regional planning. Geneva: World Health Organization, 1999.

9

At the national level

A national pandemic planning committee should be formed, including representatives from the following areas.

- Appropriate government departments (e.g. health, social services)
- Public health service
- Those responsible for licensing and quality control of vaccines
- Healthcare professionals
- Vaccine and drug manufacturers and distributors
- Health promotion and communication experts

The planning committee should ensure that both national and local pandemic plans are in place. With the emergence of a pandemic virus, it would be expected to implement these plans and co-ordinate the following.

1. Securing and controlling supplies of an effective vaccine, pneumococcal vaccine and antiviral agents and expediting licensing where necessary
2. Establishing categories of individuals to be immunized or to receive antiviral prophylaxis. This means prioritizing and quantifying because supplies may be limited
3. Planning the logistics of vaccine distribution
4. Increasing virological surveillance
5. Characterizing virus isolates, including analysis of antiviral sensitivity
6. Establishing a formal mechanism to declare a pandemic and issuing timely and authoritative advice and information at all stages to health professionals, the public and the media
7. Implementing a programme of mass vaccination when appropriate
8. Collating information on adverse reactions to vaccines and drugs

9

9. Collating epidemiological data, including information on anti-body prevalence, primary care consultation rates for defined illnesses, absenteeism, hospital activity analysis and mortality statistics
10. Collating information on the antimicrobial sensitivity of bacterial isolates from pneumonic complications of influenza and providing guidance to medical practitioners

At the local level

The following people are likely to be involved in the development of local plans.

- District and hospital health administrators
- Public health officials
- Local medical committee
- District infection control team
- Bacteriologist
- Virologist
- Epidemiologist
- Pharmacist
- Paediatrician
- Other secondary care specialists
- Hospital and community nurses
- Health-education and information officers
- Bed-bureau co-ordinator
- Immunization co-ordinator
- Representatives from social services, voluntary organizations, education, the media, emergency services and the local authority.

9

The local planning committee should ensure that contingency arrangements are in place and that, when necessary, it can carry out the following.

1. Estimating the local requirement for vaccine and antivirals
2. Identifying patients in nationally agreed priority groups and providing vaccine and antiviral prophylaxis
3. Providing vaccine and antiviral prophylaxis to essential staff
4. Disseminating information on the vaccination programme, what patients should do if they become infected and when they should call the doctor
5. Issuing and updating guidance to medical and nursing staff on the management of influenza and its complications, including the role of antivirals and antibiotics
6. Formulating contingency staffing arrangements for primary and secondary healthcare and social services to compensate for staff absences
7. Coping with large numbers of ill and dying, for example by
   - prioritizing workload in general medical practice and social services
   - increasing access to pharmacies
   - deferring non-urgent hospital admissions
   - reducing outpatient clinics
   - suspending day-care facilities
   - training temporary staff and volunteers
   - providing additional storage and disposal of bodies
8. Considering guidelines for the use of scarce resources (e.g. intensive care facilities)
9. Providing and disseminating authoritative advice to local hospitals, health professionals, the public and the media
10. Collating local information on the antimicrobial sensitivity of bacterial isolates from pneumonic complications of influenza

9

One of the few certainties of the approaching millennium is that another pandemic of influenza will occur. The events in Hong Kong in 1997 suggest that this future pandemic could cause as many millions of deaths as the Spanish influenza of 1918–1920, unless we make adequate preparations.

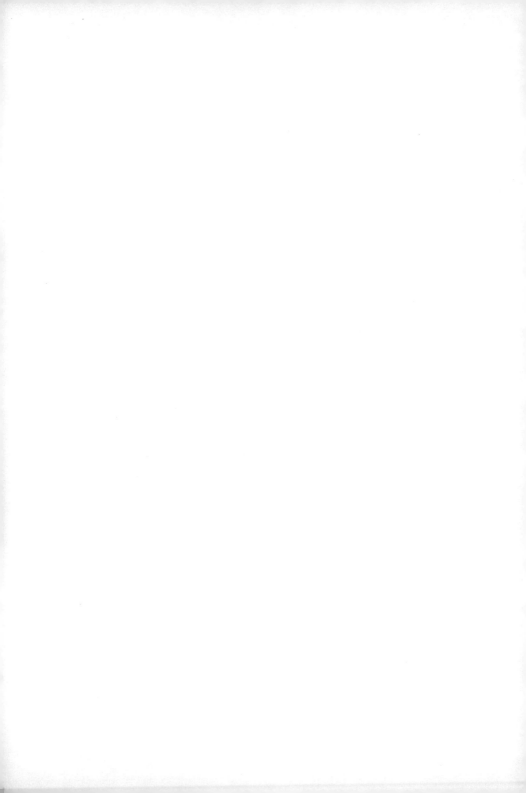